THE 2002 OFFICIAL PATIENT'S SOURCEBOOK

on

APHASIA

JAMES N. PARKER, M.D.
AND PHILIP M. PARKER, PH.D., EDITORS

D1307007

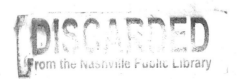

ii

ICON Health Publications
ICON Group International, Inc.
4370 La Jolla Village Drive, 4th Floor
San Diego, CA 92122 USA

Printed in the United States of America.

Last digit indicates print number: 10 9 8 7 6 4 5 3 2 1

Publisher, Health Care: Tiffany LaRochelle
Editor(s): James Parker, M.D., Philip Parker, Ph.D.

Publisher's note: The ideas, procedures, and suggestions contained in this book are not intended as a substitute for consultation with your physician. All matters regarding your health require medical supervision. As new medical or scientific information becomes available from academic and clinical research, recommended treatments and drug therapies may undergo changes. The authors, editors, and publisher have attempted to make the information in this book up to date and accurate in accord with accepted standards at the time of publication. The authors, editors, and publisher are not responsible for errors or omissions or for consequences from application of the book, and make no warranty, expressed or implied, in regard to the contents of this book. Any practice described in this book should be applied by the reader in accordance with professional standards of care used in regard to the unique circumstances that may apply in each situation, in close consultation with a qualified physician. The reader is advised to always check product information (package inserts) for changes and new information regarding dose and contraindications before taking any drug or pharmacological product. Caution is especially urged when using new or infrequently ordered drugs, herbal remedies, vitamins and supplements, alternative therapies, complementary therapies and medicines, and integrative medical treatments.

Cataloging-in-Publication Data

Parker, James N., 1961-
Parker, Philip M., 1960-

The 2002 Official Patient's Sourcebook on Aphasia: A Revised and Updated Directory for the Internet Age/James N. Parker and Philip M. Parker, editors
        p.   cm.
Includes bibliographical references, glossary and index.
ISBN: 0-597-83177-7
1. Aphasia-Popular works.   I. Title.

Disclaimer

This publication is not intended to be used for the diagnosis or treatment of a health problem or as a substitute for consultation with licensed medical professionals. It is sold with the understanding that he publisher, editors, and authors are not engaging in the rendering of medical, psychological, financial, legal, or other professional services.

References to any entity, product, service, or source of information that may be contained in this publication should not be considered an endorsement, either direct or implied, by the publisher, editors or authors. ICON Group International, Inc., the editors, or the authors are not responsible for the content of any Web pages nor publications referenced in this publication.

Copyright Notice

Dedication

To the healthcare professionals dedicating their time and efforts to the study of aphasia.

Acknowledgements

The collective knowledge generated from academic and applied research summarized in various references has been critical in the creation of this sourcebook which is best viewed as a comprehensive compilation and collection of information prepared by various official agencies which directly or indirectly are dedicated to aphasia. All of the *Official Patient's Sourcebooks* draw from various agencies and institutions associated with the United States Department of Health and Human Services, and in particular, the Office of the Secretary of Health and Human Services (OS), the Administration for Children and Families (ACF), the Administration on Aging (AOA), the Agency for Healthcare Research and Quality (AHRQ), the Agency for Toxic Substances and Disease Registry (ATSDR), the Centers for Disease Control and Prevention (CDC), the Food and Drug Administration (FDA), the Healthcare Financing Administration (HCFA), the Health Resources and Services Administration (HRSA), the Indian Health Service (IHS), the institutions of the National Institutes of Health (NIH), the Program Support Center (PSC), and the Substance Abuse and Mental Health Services Administration (SAMHSA). In addition to these sources, information gathered from the National Library of Medicine, the United States Patent Office, the European Union, and their related organizations has been invaluable in the creation of this sourcebook. Some of the work represented was financially supported by the Research and Development Committee at INSEAD. This support is gratefully acknowledged. Finally, special thanks are owed to Tiffany LaRochelle for her excellent editorial support.

About the Editors

James N. Parker, M.D.

Dr. James N. Parker received his Bachelor of Science degree in Psychobiology from the University of California, Riverside and his M.D. from the University of California, San Diego. In addition to authoring numerous research publications, he has lectured at various academic institutions. Dr. Parker is the medical editor for the *Official Patient's Sourcebook* series published by ICON Health Publications.

Philip M. Parker, Ph.D.

Philip M. Parker is the Eli Lilly Chair Professor of Innovation, Business and Society at INSEAD (Fontainebleau, France and Singapore). Dr. Parker has also been Professor at the University of California, San Diego and has taught courses at Harvard University, the Hong Kong University of Science and Technology, the Massachusetts Institute of Technology, Stanford University, and UCLA. Dr. Parker is the associate editor for the *Official Patient's Sourcebook* series published by ICON Health Publications.

About ICON Health Publications

In addition to aphasia, *Official Patient's Sourcebooks* are available for the following related topics:

- The Official Patient's Sourcebook on Dysphagia
- The Official Patient's Sourcebook on Laryngeal Papillomatosis
- The Official Patient's Sourcebook on Smell and Taste Disorders
- The Official Patient's Sourcebook on Spasmodic Dysphonia
- The Official Patient's Sourcebook on Stuttering
- The Official Patient's Sourcebook on Velocardiofacial Syndrome
- The Official Patient's Sourcebook on Vocal Abuse and Misuse
- The Official Patient's Sourcebook on Vocal Cord Paralysis

To discover more about ICON Health Publications, simply check with your preferred online booksellers, including Barnes & Noble.com and Amazon.com which currently carry all of our titles. Or, feel free to contact us directly for bulk purchases or institutional discounts:

ICON Group International, Inc.
4370 La Jolla Village Drive, Fourth Floor
San Diego, CA 92122 USA
Fax: 858-546-4341
Web site: **www.icongrouponline.com/health**

Table of Contents

INTRODUCTION

Overview

Dr. C. Everett Koop, former U.S. Surgeon General, once said, "The best prescription is knowledge."[1] The Agency for Healthcare Research and Quality (AHRQ) of the National Institutes of Health (NIH) echoes this view and recommends that every patient incorporate education into the treatment process. According to the AHRQ:

> Finding out more about your condition is a good place to start. By contacting groups that support your condition, visiting your local library, and searching on the Internet, you can find good information to help guide your treatment decisions. Some information may be hard to find — especially if you don't know where to look.[2]

As the AHRQ mentions, finding the right information is not an obvious task. Though many physicians and public officials had thought that the emergence of the Internet would do much to assist patients in obtaining reliable information, in March 2001 the National Institutes of Health issued the following warning:

> The number of Web sites offering health-related resources grows every day. Many sites provide valuable information, while others may have information that is unreliable or misleading.[3]

---

[1] Quotation from **http://www.drkoop.com**.
[2] The Agency for Healthcare Research and Quality (AHRQ):
http://www.ahcpr.gov/consumer/diaginfo.htm.
[3] From the NIH, National Cancer Institute (NCI):
http://cancertrials.nci.nih.gov/beyond/evaluating.html.

Since the late 1990s, physicians have seen a general increase in patient Internet usage rates. Patients frequently enter their doctor's offices with printed Web pages of home remedies in the guise of latest medical research. This scenario is so common that doctors often spend more time dispelling misleading information than guiding patients through sound therapies. *The Official Patient's Sourcebook on Aphasia* has been created for patients who have decided to make education and research an integral part of the treatment process. The pages that follow will tell you where and how to look for information covering virtually all topics related to aphasia, from the essentials to the most advanced areas of research.

The title of this book includes the word "official." This reflects the fact that the sourcebook draws from public, academic, government, and peer-reviewed research. Selected readings from various agencies are reproduced to give you some of the latest official information available to date on aphasia.

Given patients' increasing sophistication in using the Internet, abundant references to reliable Internet-based resources are provided throughout this sourcebook. Where possible, guidance is provided on how to obtain free-of-charge, primary research results as well as more detailed information via the Internet. E-book and electronic versions of this sourcebook are fully interactive with each of the Internet sites mentioned (clicking on a hyperlink automatically opens your browser to the site indicated). Hard copy users of this sourcebook can type cited Web addresses directly into their browsers to obtain access to the corresponding sites. Since we are working with ICON Health Publications, hard copy *Sourcebooks* are frequently updated and printed on demand to ensure that the information provided is current.

In addition to extensive references accessible via the Internet, every chapter presents a "Vocabulary Builder." Many health guides offer glossaries of technical or uncommon terms in an appendix. In editing this sourcebook, we have decided to place a smaller glossary within each chapter that covers terms used in that chapter. Given the technical nature of some chapters, you may need to revisit many sections. Building one's vocabulary of medical terms in such a gradual manner has been shown to improve the learning process.

We must emphasize that no sourcebook on aphasia should affirm that a specific diagnostic procedure or treatment discussed in a research study, patent, or doctoral dissertation is "correct" or your best option. This sourcebook is no exception. Each patient is unique. Deciding on appropriate options is always up to the patient in consultation with their physician and healthcare providers.

Organization

This sourcebook is organized into three parts. Part I explores basic techniques to researching aphasia (e.g. finding guidelines on diagnosis, treatments, and prognosis), followed by a number of topics, including information on how to get in touch with organizations, associations, or other patient networks dedicated to aphasia. It also gives you sources of information that can help you find a doctor in your local area specializing in treating aphasia. Collectively, the material presented in Part I is a complete primer on basic research topics for patients with aphasia.

Part II moves on to advanced research dedicated to aphasia. Part II is intended for those willing to invest many hours of hard work and study. It is here that we direct you to the latest scientific and applied research on aphasia. When possible, contact names, links via the Internet, and summaries are provided. It is in Part II where the vocabulary process becomes important as authors publishing advanced research frequently use highly specialized language. In general, every attempt is made to recommend "free-to-use" options.

Part III provides appendices of useful background reading for all patients with aphasia or related disorders. The appendices are dedicated to more pragmatic issues faced by many patients with aphasia. Accessing materials via medical libraries may be the only option for some readers, so a guide is provided for finding local medical libraries which are open to the public. Part III, therefore, focuses on advice that goes beyond the biological and scientific issues facing patients with aphasia.

Scope

While this sourcebook covers aphasia, your doctor, research publications, and specialists may refer to your condition using a variety of terms. Therefore, you should understand that aphasia is often considered a synonym or a condition closely related to the following:

- Acquired Aphasia with Convulsive Disorder

- Acquired Epileptic Aphasia

- Infantile Acquired Aphasia

In addition to synonyms and related conditions, physicians may refer to aphasia using certain coding systems. The International Classification of Diseases, 9th Revision, Clinical Modification (ICD-9-CM) is the most commonly used system of classification for the world's illnesses. Your physician may use this coding system as an administrative or tracking tool. The following classification is commonly used for aphasia:[4]

- 315.31 developmental language disorder

- 438.11 aphasia

- 784.3 aphasia

For the purposes of this sourcebook, we have attempted to be as inclusive as possible, looking for official information for all of the synonyms relevant to aphasia. You may find it useful to refer to synonyms when accessing databases or interacting with healthcare professionals and medical librarians.

Moving Forward

Since the 1980s, the world has seen a proliferation of healthcare guides covering most illnesses. Some are written by patients or their family members. These generally take a layperson's approach to understanding and coping with an illness or disorder. They can be uplifting, encouraging, and highly supportive. Other guides are authored by physicians or other healthcare providers who have a more clinical outlook. Each of these two styles of guide has its purpose and can be quite useful.

As editors, we have chosen a third route. We have chosen to expose you to as many sources of official and peer-reviewed information as practical, for the purpose of educating you about basic and advanced knowledge as recognized by medical science today. You can think of this sourcebook as your personal Internet age reference librarian.

Why "Internet age"? All too often, patients diagnosed with aphasia will log on to the Internet, type words into a search engine, and receive several Web site listings which are mostly irrelevant or redundant. These patients are left to wonder where the relevant information is, and how to obtain it. Since only

---

[4] This list is based on the official version of the World Health Organization's 9th Revision, International Classification of Diseases (ICD-9). According to the National Technical Information Service, "ICD-9CM extensions, interpretations, modifications, addenda, or errata other than those approved by the U.S. Public Health Service and the Health Care Financing Administration are not to be considered official and should not be utilized. Continuous maintenance of the ICD-9-CM is the responsibility of the federal government."

the smallest fraction of information dealing with aphasia is even indexed in search engines, a non-systematic approach often leads to frustration and disappointment. With this sourcebook, we hope to direct you to the information you need that you would not likely find using popular Web directories. Beyond Web listings, in many cases we will reproduce brief summaries or abstracts of available reference materials. These abstracts often contain distilled information on topics of discussion.

While we focus on the more scientific aspects of aphasia, there is, of course, the emotional side to consider. Later in the sourcebook, we provide a chapter dedicated to helping you find peer groups and associations that can provide additional support beyond research produced by medical science. We hope that the choices we have made give you the most options available in moving forward. In this way, we wish you the best in your efforts to incorporate this educational approach into your treatment plan.

The Editors

PART I: THE ESSENTIALS

ABOUT PART I

Part I has been edited to give you access to what we feel are "the essentials" on aphasia. The essentials of a disease typically include the definition or description of the disease, a discussion of who it affects, the signs or symptoms associated with the disease, tests or diagnostic procedures that might be specific to the disease, and treatments for the disease. Your doctor or healthcare provider may have already explained the essentials of aphasia to you or even given you a pamphlet or brochure describing aphasia. Now you are searching for more in-depth information. As editors, we have decided, nevertheless, to include a discussion on where to find essential information that can complement what your doctor has already told you. In this section we recommend a process, not a particular Web site or reference book. The process ensures that, as you search the Web, you gain background information in such a way as to maximize your understanding.

CHAPTER 1. THE ESSENTIALS ON APHASIA: GUIDELINES

Overview

Official agencies, as well as federally-funded institutions supported by national grants, frequently publish a variety of guidelines on aphasia. These are typically called "Fact Sheets" or "Guidelines." They can take the form of a brochure, information kit, pamphlet, or flyer. Often they are only a few pages in length. The great advantage of guidelines over other sources is that they are often written with the patient in mind. Since new guidelines on aphasia can appear at any moment and be published by a number of sources, the best approach to finding guidelines is to systematically scan the Internet-based services that post them.

The National Institutes of Health (NIH)[5]

The National Institutes of Health (NIH) is the first place to search for relatively current patient guidelines and fact sheets on aphasia. Originally founded in 1887, the NIH is one of the world's foremost medical research centers and the federal focal point for medical research in the United States. At any given time, the NIH supports some 35,000 research grants at universities, medical schools, and other research and training institutions, both nationally and internationally. The rosters of those who have conducted research or who have received NIH support over the years include the world's most illustrious scientists and physicians. Among them are 97 scientists who have won the Nobel Prize for achievement in medicine.

---

[5] Adapted from the NIH: **http://www.nih.gov/about/NIHoverview.html**.

There is no guarantee that any one Institute will have a guideline on a specific disease, though the National Institutes of Health collectively publish over 600 guidelines for both common and rare diseases. The best way to access NIH guidelines is via the Internet. Although the NIH is organized into many different Institutes and Offices, the following is a list of key Web sites where you are most likely to find NIH clinical guidelines and publications dealing with aphasia and associated conditions:

- Office of the Director (OD); guidelines consolidated across agencies available at **http://www.nih.gov/health/consumer/conkey.htm**

- National Library of Medicine (NLM); extensive encyclopedia (A.D.A.M., Inc.) with guidelines available at **http://www.nlm.nih.gov/medlineplus/healthtopics.html**

- National Institute on Deafness and Other Communication Disorders (NIDCD); fact sheets and guidelines available at **http://www.nidcd.nih.gov/health/health.htm**

Among the above, the National Institute on Deafness and Other Communication Disorders (NIDCD) is particularly noteworthy. The mission of the NIDCD is to conduct and support biomedical and behavioral research and research training in the normal and disordered processes of hearing, balance, smell, taste, voice, speech, and language.[6] The Institute also conducts and supports research and research training related to disease prevention and health promotion; addresses special biomedical and behavioral problems associated with people who have communication impairments or disorders; and supports efforts to create devices which substitute for lost and impaired sensory and communication function.

The following patient guideline was recently published by the NIDCD on aphasia.

What Is Aphasia?[7]

Aphasia is a language disorder that results from damage to portions of the brain that are responsible for language. For most people, these are parts of the left side (hemisphere) of the brain. Aphasia usually occurs suddenly, often as the result of a stroke or head injury, but it may also develop slowly,

---

[6] This paragraph has been adapted from the NIDCD: **http://www.nidcd.nih.gov/about/about.htm**. "Adapted" signifies that a passage has been reproduced exactly or slightly edited for this book.

[7] Adapted from the National Institute on Deafness and Other Communication Disorders (NIDCD): **http://www.nidcd.nih.gov/health/pubs_vsl/aphasia.htm**.

as in the case of a brain tumor. The disorder impairs both the expression and understanding of language as well as reading and writing. Aphasia may co-occur with speech disorders such as dysarthria or apraxia of speech, which also result from brain damage.

Who Has Aphasia?

Anyone can acquire aphasia, but most people who have aphasia are in their middle to late years. Men and women are equally affected. It is estimated that approximately 80,000 individuals acquire aphasia each year. About one million persons in the United States currently have aphasia.

What Causes Aphasia?

Aphasia is caused by damage to one or more of the language areas of the brain. Many times, the cause of the brain injury is a stroke. A stroke occurs when, for some reason, blood is unable to reach a part of the brain. Brain cells die when they do not receive their normal supply of blood, which carries oxygen and important nutrients. Other causes of brain injury are severe blows to the head, brain tumors, brain infections, and other conditions of the brain.

Individuals with Broca's aphasia have damage to the frontal lobe of the brain. These individuals frequently speak in short, meaningful phrases that are produced with great effort. Broca's aphasia is thus characterized as a nonfluent aphasia. Affected people often omit small words such as "is," "and," and "the." For example, a person with Broca's aphasia may say, "Walk dog" meaning, "I will take the dog for a walk." The same sentence could also mean "You take the dog for a walk," or "The dog walked out of the yard," depending on the circumstances. Individuals with Broca's aphasia are able to understand the speech of others to varying degrees. Because of this, they are often aware of their difficulties and can become easily frustrated by their speaking problems. Individuals with Broca's aphasia often have right-sided weakness or paralysis of the arm and leg because the frontal lobe is also important for body movement.

In contrast to Broca's aphasia, damage to the temporal lobe may result in a fluent aphasia that is called Wernicke's aphasia. Individuals with Wernicke's aphasia may speak in long sentences that have no meaning, add unnecessary words, and even create new "words." For example, someone with

Wernicke's aphasia may say, "You know that smoodle pinkered and that I want to get him round and take care of him like you want before," meaning "The dog needs to go out so I will take him for a walk." Individuals with Wernicke's aphasia usually have great difficulty understanding speech and are therefore often unaware of their mistakes. These individuals usually have no body weakness because their brain injury is not near the parts of the brain that control movement.

A third type of aphasia, global aphasia, results from damage to extensive portions of the language areas of the brain. Individuals with global aphasia have severe communication difficulties and may be extremely limited in their ability to speak or comprehend language.

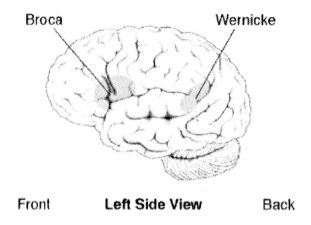

Broca   Wernicke

Front   Left Side View   Back

How Is Aphasia Diagnosed?

Aphasia is usually first recognized by the physician who treats the individual for his or her brain injury. Frequently this is a neurologist. The physician typically performs tests that require the individual to follow commands, answer questions, name objects, and converse. If the physician suspects aphasia, the individual is often referred to a speech-language pathologist, who performs a comprehensive examination of the person's ability to understand, speak, read, and write.

How Is Aphasia Treated?

In some instances an individual will completely recover from aphasia without treatment. This type of "spontaneous recovery" usually occurs following a transient ischemic attack (TIA), a kind of stroke in which the blood flow to the brain is temporarily interrupted but quickly restored. In these circumstances, language abilities may return in a few hours or a few days. For most cases of aphasia, however, language recovery is not as quick or as complete. While many individuals with aphasia also experience a period of partial spontaneous recovery (in which some language abilities return over a period of a few days to a month after the brain injury), some amount of aphasia typically remains. In these instances, speech-language therapy is often helpful. Recovery usually continues over a 2-year period. Most people believe that the most effective treatment begins early in the recovery process. Some of the factors that influence the amount of improvement include the cause of the brain damage, the area of the brain that was damaged, the extent of the brain injury, and the age and health of the individual. Additional factors include motivation, handedness, and educational level.

Aphasia therapy strives to improve an individual's ability to communicate by helping the person to use remaining abilities, to restore language abilities as much as possible, to compensate for language problems, and to learn other methods of communicating. Treatment may be offered in individual or group settings. Individual therapy focuses on the specific needs of the person. Group therapy offers the opportunity to use new communication skills in a comfortable setting. Stroke clubs, which are regional support groups formed by individuals who have had a stroke, are available in most major cities. These clubs also offer the opportunity for individuals with aphasia to try new communication skills. In addition, stroke clubs can help the individual and his or her family adjust to the life changes that accompany stroke and aphasia. Family involvement is often a crucial component of aphasia treatment so that family members can learn the best way to communicate with their loved one.

Family members are encouraged to:

- Simplify language by using short, uncomplicated sentences.

- Repeat the content words or write down key words to clarify meaning as needed.

- Maintain a natural conversational manner appropriate for an adult.

- Minimize distractions, such as a blaring radio, whenever possible.

- Include the person with aphasia in conversations.

- Ask for and value the opinion of the person with aphasia, especially regarding family matters.

- Encourage any type of communication, whether it is speech, gesture, pointing, or drawing.

- Avoid correcting the individual's speech.

- Allow the individual plenty of time to talk.

- Help the individual become involved outside the home. Seek out support groups such as stroke clubs.

What Research Is Being Done for Aphasia?

Aphasia research is exploring new ways to evaluate and treat aphasia as well as to further understanding of the function of the brain. Brain imaging techniques are helping to define brain function, determine the severity of brain damage, and predict the severity of the aphasia. These procedures include PET (positron emission tomography), CT (computed tomography), and MRI (magnetic resonance imaging) as well as the new functional magnetic resonance (fMRI), which identifies areas of the brain that are used during activities such as speaking or listening. In-depth testing of the language ability of individuals with the various aphasic syndromes is helping to design effective treatment strategies. The use of computers in aphasia treatment is being studied. Promising new drugs administered shortly after some types of stroke are being investigated as ways to reduce the severity of aphasia.

Where Can I Get Additional Information?

For more information on aphasia, contact:

American Academy of Neurology
1080 Montreal Avenue
St. Paul, MN 55116
Voice: (651) 695-1940
Internet: **www.aan.com**

American Heart Association
7272 Greenville Avenue
Dallas, TX 75231
Voice: (800) 242-8721
Internet: **www.americanheart.org**

American Speech-Language-Hearing Association
10801 Rockville Pike
Rockville, MD 20852
Voice/TTY: (301) 897-5700
Voice: (800) 638-8255
Internet: **www.asha.org**

Brain Injury Association, Inc.
105 North Alfred Street
Alexandria, VA 22314
Voice: (800) 444-6443
Internet: **www.biausa.org**

Easter Seals
230 West Monroe, Suite 1800
Chicago, IL 60606
Voice: (800) 221-6827
Internet: **www.easter-seals.org**

National Aphasia Association
156 Fifth Avenue, Suite 707
New York, NY 10010
Voice: (800) 922-4622
Internet: **www.aphasia.org**

National Stroke Association
9707 East Easter Lane
Englewood, CO 80112-3747
Voice: (800) 787-6537
Internet: **www.stroke.org**

More Guideline Sources

The guideline above on aphasia is only one example of the kind of material that you can find online and free of charge. The remainder of this chapter will direct you to other sources which either publish or can help you find additional guidelines on topics related to aphasia. Many of the guidelines listed below address topics that may be of particular relevance to your specific situation or of special interest to only some patients with aphasia. Due to space limitations these sources are listed in a concise manner. Do not hesitate to consult the following sources by either using the Internet hyperlink provided, or, in cases where the contact information is provided, contacting the publisher or author directly.

Topic Pages: MEDLINEplus

For patients wishing to go beyond guidelines published by specific Institutes of the NIH, the National Library of Medicine has created a vast and patient-oriented healthcare information portal called MEDLINEplus. Within this Internet-based system are "health topic pages." You can think of a health topic page as a guide to patient guides. To access this system, log on to **http://www.nlm.nih.gov/medlineplus/healthtopics.html**. From there you can either search using the alphabetical index or browse by broad topic areas. Recently, MEDLINEplus listed the following as being relevant to aphasia:

- Guides On aphasia

    Aphasia
    http://www.nlm.nih.gov/medlineplus/aphasia.html

- Guides on Human Anatomy and Systems

    Brain and Nervous System Topics
    http://www.nlm.nih.gov/medlineplus/brainandnervoussystem.html

- Other Guides

    Stroke
    http://www.nlm.nih.gov/medlineplus/stroke.html

    Speech & Communication Disorders
    http://www.nlm.nih.gov/medlineplus/speechcommunicationdisorders.html

    Stroke
    http://www.nlm.nih.gov/medlineplus/ency/article/000726.htm

    Pick's disease
    http://www.nlm.nih.gov/medlineplus/ency/article/000744.htm

    Mental status tests
    http://www.nlm.nih.gov/medlineplus/ency/article/003326.htm

    Dementia
    http://www.nlm.nih.gov/medlineplus/ency/article/000739.htm

Hemorrhagic stroke
http://www.nlm.nih.gov/medlineplus/ency/article/000761.htm

Brain abscess
http://www.nlm.nih.gov/medlineplus/ency/article/000783.htm

Multi-infarct dementia
http://www.nlm.nih.gov/medlineplus/ency/article/000746.htm

General paresis
http://www.nlm.nih.gov/medlineplus/ency/article/000748.htm

Stroke secondary to atherosclerosis
http://www.nlm.nih.gov/medlineplus/ency/article/000738.htm

Stroke secondary to cardiogenic embolism
http://www.nlm.nih.gov/medlineplus/ency/article/000735.htm

Stroke secondary to syphilis
http://www.nlm.nih.gov/medlineplus/ency/article/000728.htm

Stroke secondary to carotid dissection
http://www.nlm.nih.gov/medlineplus/ency/article/000732.htm

Within the health topic page dedicated to aphasia, the following was recently recommended to patients:

- General/Overviews

  Aphasia
  Source: American Speech-Language-Hearing Association
  http://www.asha.org/speech/disabilities/Aphasia_1.cfm

  Aphasia
  Source: National Aphasia Association
  http://www.aphasia.org/NAAfactsheet.html

- Coping

  Communicating with Someone Who Has Had a Stroke
  Source: Mayo Foundation for Medical Education and Research
  http://www.mayoclinic.com/invoke.cfm?id=HQ00659

  Family Adjustment to Aphasia
  Source: American Speech-Language-Hearing Association
  http://www.asha.org/speech/disabilities/Family-Adjustment-to-Aphasia.cfm

- Specific Conditions/Aspects

  Understanding Primary Progressive Aphasia
  Source: National Aphasia Association
  http://www.aphasia.org/NAAppa.html

- Children

  Landau-Kleffner Syndrome
  Source: National Institute on Deafness and Other Communication Disorders
  http://www.nidcd.nih.gov/health/pubs_vsl/landklfs.htm

  Landau-Kleffner Syndrome
  Source: img src='/medlineplus/images/shortsummary.gif' width='90' height='17' border=0 alt='Short Summary'> (National Institute of Neurological Disorders and Stroke
  http://www.ninds.nih.gov/health_and_medical/disorders/landaukleffnersyndrome_doc.htm

- From the National Institutes of Health

  Aphasia
  Source: National Institute on Deafness and Other Communication Disorders
  http://www.nidcd.nih.gov/health/pubs_vsl/aphasia.htm

  Aphasia
  Source: img src='/medlineplus/images/shortsummary.gif' width='90' height='17' border=0 alt='Short Summary'> (National Institute of Neurological Disorders and Stroke
  http://www.ninds.nih.gov/health_and_medical/disorders/aphasia.htm

- Law and Policy

  Employment Rights of People with Communication Disabilities
  Source: American Speech-Language-Hearing Association
  http://www.asha.org/takeaction/Employment-Rights-of-People-with-Communication-Disabilities.cfm

- Lists of Print Publications

  Selected Readings Appropriate for Individuals with Aphasia, Their Families, and Professionals
  Source: National Aphasia Association
  http://www.aphasia.org/NAAreadings.html

  Selected Readings on Psychosocial Aspects of Aphasia
  Source: National Aphasia Association
  http://www.aphasia.org/NAApsychosocial_readings.html

- Organizations

  American Speech-Language-Hearing Association
  http://www.asha.org

  National Aphasia Association
  http://www.aphasia.org

  National Institute of Neurological Disorders and Stroke
  http://www.ninds.nih.gov/

  National Institute on Deafness and Other Communication Disorders
  http://www.nidcd.nih.gov/

- Research

  Adult Aphasia: Recent Research
  Source: National Institute on Deafness and Other Communication Disorders
  http://www.nidcd.nih.gov/health/pubs_vsl/adultaphasia.htm

  Aphasia Therapy Research - Annual Update
  Source: National Aphasia Association
  http://www.aphasia.org/newsletter/121aphasiatherapy.html

If you do not find topics of interest when browsing health topic pages, then you can choose to use the advanced search utility of MEDLINEplus at **http://www.nlm.nih.gov/medlineplus/advancedsearch.html**. This utility is similar to the NIH Search Utility, with the exception that it only includes material linked within the MEDLINEplus system (mostly patient-oriented information). It also has the disadvantage of generating unstructured results. We recommend, therefore, that you use this method only if you have a very targeted search.

The Combined Health Information Database (CHID)

CHID Online is a reference tool that maintains a database directory of thousands of journal articles and patient education guidelines on aphasia and related conditions. One of the advantages of CHID over other sources is that it offers summaries that describe the guidelines available, including contact information and pricing. CHID's general Web site is **http://chid.nih.gov/**. To search this database, go to **http://chid.nih.gov/detail/detail.html**. In particular, you can use the advanced search options to look up pamphlets, reports, brochures, and information kits. The following was recently posted in this archive:

- **Aphasia: Understanding This Language Problem**

  Source: San Bruno, CA: Krames Communications. 1997. [4 p.].

  Contact: Available from Krames Communications. 1100 Grundy Lane, San Bruno, CA 94066-3030. (800) 333-3032. PRICE: Single copy free; bulk rates available.

  Summary: This brochure presents a basic description of aphasia, a loss of language skills that may occur if the brain is damaged by injury or illness. The brochure first defines aphasia and lists the common symptoms of the condition. Other topics include the role of the speech therapist in diagnosing and treating aphasia, testing word use, setting goals for speech rehabilitation, the role of the family, and related problems including dysarthria (lose of control of some muscles in the face and mouth) and dysphagia (swallowing difficulties). One sidebar outlines recommendations for family and friends who wish to help a patient with recovery. The brochure is illustrated with full-color line drawings. 4 figures.

- **Adult Has Aphasia: For the Family: The Management and Treatment of the Patient With Aphasia. 5th ed**

  Source: Austin, TX: Pro-Ed. 1995. 32 p.

  Contact: Available from Pro-Ed. 8700 Shoal Creek Boulevard, Austin, TX 78757. (512) 451-3246; Fax (512) 451-8542. PRICE: $6.00 each; $49.00 for package of 10. Item Number 6925 (single copy); Item Number 6926 (package of 10).

  Summary: The families of people with aphasia play a vital role in their recovery. This booklet is written to help families and patients alike understand some of the problems surrounding aphasia. Aphasia is defined as an impairment in language ability after an injury to the brain. The booklet defines aphasia, then discusses the causes of aphasia, the kinds of aphasia, patient-family interactions, physical disabilities, personality changes, a comprehensive treatment program, and speech and language retraining. A final chapter presents a list of recommendations for family members. The author provides practical suggestions for everyday interactions between people with aphasia and their families.

- **Adult Aphasia: Understanding the Disability**

  Source: Cambridge, MA: Department of Communication Disorders, Youville Hospital and Rehabilitation Center. 1994. 12 p.

  Contact: Available from Youville Hospital and Rehabilitation Center. Department of Communication Disorders, 1575 Cambridge Street, Cambridge, MA 02138-4398. (617) 876-4344. PRICE: $4.00 each.

  Summary: This manual helps family members and caregivers understand adult aphasia, a language disability that is often the result of a stroke (cerebrovascular accident or CVA). The manual reminds readers that each individual's recovery will vary, depending on the severity of the stroke and other factors. The manual provides definitions of related terms and then discusses aphasia and its impact on expression and understanding. The authors then discuss complications, including factors that may affect the communication interaction, sensation loss, and visual field cuts. A lengthy section provides suggestions for helping the patient to remain a person and stay involved in his or her own health care. Additional sections address loss of independence, automatic (non-propositional) speech, emotional lability, the time commitments required for effective communication, perseveration, interpersonal relationships, and medical follow ups. The manual concludes with a question and answer section. Comments from patients and caregivers are included throughout the text. 3 figures. 2 references. (AA-M).

- **Aphasia: A Guide for the Patient and Family**

  Source: Stow, OH: Interactive Therapeutics, Inc. 1993. 53 p.

  Contact: Available from Interactive Therapeutics, Inc. P.O. Box 1805, Stow, OH 44224. (800) 253-5111 or (216) 688-1371; Fax (330) 923-3030; E-mail: winteract@aol.com. PRICE: $4.50 each for 1 to 25 copies; bulk rates available.

  Summary: This patient education booklet describes aphasia, a loss or reduction of language skills due to brain injury. The booklet presents information in eleven chapters: brain function, causes, definitions of aphasia, accompanying problems, treatment options, self-care and family participation in care, community support options, common questions and answers, and spare time activities. The booklet concludes with a glossary and a list of recommended resources for additional reading.

- **American Speech-Language-Hearing Association Answers Questions About Adult Aphasia**

  Source: Rockville, MD: American Speech-Language-Hearing Association (ASHA). 199x. (2 p.).

  Contact: Available from American Speech-Language-Hearing Association (ASHA). Product Sales, 10801 Rockville Pike, Rockville, MD 20852. (888) 498-6699. TTY (301) 897-0157. Website: www.asha.org. PRICE: Single copy free; bulk orders available. Item Number 0210114.

  Summary: This brochure provides basic information about adult aphasia. Aphasia is defined as a condition in which an individual has difficulty expressing thoughts and understanding what is said or written by others. The brochure, written in question and answer format, covers some of the language problems associated with aphasia, why it takes a person with aphasia so long to respond, swearing in individuals with aphasia, related communication problems caused by stroke or head injury, some of the physical problems connected with brain damage, spontaneous recovery, and support available for the person with aphasia. The brochure stresses both the importance of seeking therapy from a speech-language pathologist and the vital role that family and friends can play in rehabilitation. The brochure includes the toll-free telephone number of the American Speech-Language-Hearing Association (800-638-8255).

- **[National Aphasia Association Brochure]**

  Source: New York, NY: National Aphasia Association. 199x. [8 p.].

  Contact: Available from National Aphasia Association Response Center. 351 Butternut Court, Millersville, MD 21108. (800) 922-4622. Fax (410) 729-5724. Website: www.aphasia.org. PRICE: $1.00 plus shipping and handling.

  Summary: This brochure depicts the daily struggles of coping with aphasia, a disorder of communication that results from various kinds of damage to the brain and impairs a person's ability to speak, comprehend speech, and possibly to read and write. The brochure notes that aphasia can occur at any age and most often is the result of a stroke. Because of the communication difficulty, people with aphasia are socially isolated and in need of programs to improve the quality of their lives. The brochure is written in large print and includes black and white photographs of a variety of people with aphasia. The brochure is designed to raise public awareness of aphasia and to raise funds for the

National Aphasia Association (NAA). The last two pages of the brochure describe the NAA, an organization dedicated to promoting the care and rehabilitation of people with aphasia through public education, encouragement of the nationwide Aphasia Community Group network, and support of research. The toll free phone number (800-922-4622) of the association is included, as is a form with which readers can send financial support to the organization.

The National Guideline Clearinghouse™

The National Guideline Clearinghouse™ offers hundreds of evidence-based clinical practice guidelines published in the United States and other countries. You can search their site located at **http://www.guideline.gov** by using the keyword "aphasia" or synonyms. The following was recently posted:

- **Evaluation of surgery for Parkinson's disease. A report of the Therapeutics and Technology Assessment Subcommittee of the American Academy of Neurology. The Task Force on Surgery for Parkinson's Disease.**

  Source: American Academy of Neurology.; 1999 December; 12 pages

  http://www.guideline.gov/FRAMESETS/guideline_fs.asp?guideline=002056&sSearch_string=aphasia

- **Practice parameters for the assessment and treatment of children and adolescents with language and learning disorders.**

  Source: American Academy of Child and Adolescent Psychiatry.; 1998; 17 pages

  http://www.guideline.gov/FRAMESETS/guideline_fs.asp?guideline=000756&sSearch_string=aphasia

Healthfinder™

Healthfinder™ is an additional source sponsored by the U.S. Department of Health and Human Services which offers links to hundreds of other sites that contain healthcare information. This Web site is located at **http://www.healthfinder.gov**. Again, keyword searches can be used to find guidelines. The following was recently found in this database:

- **Adult Aphasia: Recent Research**

  Summary: This consumer health education brochure provides basic information about aphasia, a language disorder that results from damage to portions of the brain that are responsible for language.

  Source: National Institute on Deafness and Other Communication Disorders Information Clearinghouse

  http://www.healthfinder.gov/scripts/recordpass.asp?RecordType=0&RecordID=31

The NIH Search Utility

After browsing the references listed at the beginning of this chapter, you may want to explore the NIH Search Utility. This allows you to search for documents on over 100 selected Web sites that comprise the NIH-WEB-SPACE. Each of these servers is "crawled" and indexed on an ongoing basis. Your search will produce a list of various documents, all of which will relate in some way to aphasia. The drawbacks of this approach are that the information is not organized by theme and that the references are often a mix of information for professionals and patients. Nevertheless, a large number of the listed Web sites provide useful background information. We can only recommend this route, therefore, for relatively rare or specific disorders, or when using highly targeted searches. To use the NIH search utility, visit the following Web page: **http://search.nih.gov/index.html**.

Additional Web Sources

A number of Web sites that often link to government sites are available to the public. These can also point you in the direction of essential information. The following is a representative sample:

- AOL: **http://search.aol.com/cat.adp?id=168&layer=&from=subcats**

- drkoop.com®: **http://www.drkoop.com/conditions/ency/index.html**

- Family Village: **http://www.familyvillage.wisc.edu/specific.htm**

- Google:
  http://directory.google.com/Top/Health/Conditions_and_Diseases/

- Med Help International: **http://www.medhelp.org/HealthTopics/A.html**

- Open Directory Project:
  http://dmoz.org/Health/Conditions_and_Diseases/

- Yahoo.com: **http://dir.yahoo.com/Health/Diseases_and_Conditions/**
- WebMD®Health: **http://my.webmd.com/health_topics**

Vocabulary Builder

The material in this chapter may have contained a number of unfamiliar words. The following Vocabulary Builder introduces you to terms used in this chapter that have not been covered in the previous chapter:

Aphasia: Defect or loss of the power of expression by speech, writing, or signs, or of comprehending spoken or written language, due to injury or disease of the brain centres. [EU]

Cardiogenic: Originating in the heart; caused by abnormal function of the heart. [EU]

Cerebrovascular: Pertaining to the blood vessels of the cerebrum, or brain. [EU]

Dementia: An acquired organic mental disorder with loss of intellectual abilities of sufficient severity to interfere with social or occupational functioning. The dysfunction is multifaceted and involves memory, behavior, personality, judgment, attention, spatial relations, language, abstract thought, and other executive functions. The intellectual decline is usually progressive, and initially spares the level of consciousness. [NIH]

Dysarthria: Imperfect articulation of speech due to disturbances of muscular control which result from damage to the central or peripheral nervous system. [EU]

Dysphagia: Difficulty in swallowing. [EU]

Lobe: A more or less well-defined portion of any organ, especially of the brain, lungs, and glands. Lobes are demarcated by fissures, sulci, connective tissue, and by their shape. [EU]

Neurology: A medical specialty concerned with the study of the structures, functions, and diseases of the nervous system. [NIH]

Paralysis: Loss or impairment of motor function in a part due to lesion of the neural or muscular mechanism; also by analogy, impairment of sensory function (sensory paralysis). In addition to the types named below, paralysis is further distinguished as traumatic, syphilitic, toxic, etc., according to its cause; or as obturator, ulnar, etc., according to the nerve part, or muscle specially affected. [EU]

Tomography: The recording of internal body images at a predetermined plane by means of the tomograph; called also body section roentgenography.

CHAPTER 2. SEEKING GUIDANCE

Overview

Some patients are comforted by the knowledge that a number of organizations dedicate their resources to helping people with aphasia. These associations can become invaluable sources of information and advice. Many associations offer aftercare support, financial assistance, and other important services. Furthermore, healthcare research has shown that support groups often help people to better cope with their conditions.[8] In addition to support groups, your physician can be a valuable source of guidance and support. Therefore, finding a physician that can work with your unique situation is a very important aspect of your care.

In this chapter, we direct you to resources that can help you find patient organizations and medical specialists. We begin by describing how to find associations and peer groups that can help you better understand and cope with aphasia. The chapter ends with a discussion on how to find a doctor that is right for you.

Associations and Aphasia

As mentioned by the Agency for Healthcare Research and Quality, sometimes the emotional side of an illness can be as taxing as the physical side.[9] You may have fears or feel overwhelmed by your situation. Everyone has different ways of dealing with disease or physical injury. Your attitude, your expectations, and how well you cope with your condition can all

---

[8] Churches, synagogues, and other houses of worship might also have groups that can offer you the social support you need.

[9] This section has been adapted from **http://www.ahcpr.gov/consumer/diaginf5.htm**.

influence your well-being. This is true for both minor conditions and serious illnesses. For example, a study on female breast cancer survivors revealed that women who participated in support groups lived longer and experienced better quality of life when compared with women who did not participate. In the support group, women learned coping skills and had the opportunity to share their feelings with other women in the same situation.

In addition to associations or groups that your doctor might recommend, we suggest that you consider the following list (if there is a fee for an association, you may want to check with your insurance provider to find out if the cost will be covered):

- **C.A.N.D.L.E**

  Address: C.A.N.D.L.E. 4414 McCampbell Drive, Montgomery, AL 36106

  Telephone: (334) 281-7179 Toll-free: (800) 922- 4622

  Fax: (334) 271-394

  Background: C.A.N.D.L.E. is an international not-for-profit voluntary support organization composed of parents, families, professionals, and friends of children with neurological disorders. C.A.N.D.L.E. provides educational and medical information and recommendations about all aspects of Childhood Aphasia, Autism, Pervasive Development Disorder, Landau-Kleffner Syndrome, and Epilepsy. The organization's primary focus is to act as a clearinghouse for information on childhood neurological disorders. To this end, the organization accumulates and disseminates information about these neurological disorders. It stimulates increased access to resources, answers questions from parents and professionals concerning identification, evaluation, treatment, and rehabilitation, and encourages scientific research into the causes, control, and cure of such disorders. In addition, C.A.N.D.L.E. seeks to aid parents in understanding treatment options and offer support by listening, sharing experiences, and networking families with similar disorders. Educational materials produced by the organization include brochures, journals, and a regular newsletter.

- **National Aphasia Association**

  Address: National Aphasia Association 156 Fifth Avenue, Suite 707, New York, NY 10010

  Telephone: Toll-free: (800) 922- 4622

  Fax: (212) 989-7777

  Email: Klein@aphasia.org

  Web Site: http://www.aphasia.or

Background: The National Aphasia Association is a not-for-profit organization dedicated to increasing public awareness of aphasia and other communication disorders and aiding persons with aphasia and their families. Aphasia is a neurological condition caused by damage to the left hemisphere of the brain in which communication and/or language skills (speaking, reading, writing, and comprehending others) are impaired. Established in 1987, the Association's activities include sponsoring support groups, promoting advocacy and legislative programs, supporting ongoing medical research, and maintaining an informational Web site. Other activities include support of a Response Center reachable at (800) 922-4622, publication of a biannual newsletter, sponsorship of biannual national gatherings, and production of fact sheets, reading lists and national listings of community-based support groups, and contact information for a national network of health care professionals who volunteer to respond to families in their area about local resources. A Young People's Network puts families in touch with one another for the purpose of peer support and information exchange.

Relevant area(s) of interest: Aphasia

Finding More Associations

There are a number of directories that list additional medical associations that you may find useful. While not all of these directories will provide different information than what is listed above, by consulting all of them, you will have nearly exhausted all sources for patient associations.

The National Health Information Center (NHIC)

The National Health Information Center (NHIC) offers a free referral service to help people find organizations that provide information about aphasia. For more information, see the NHIC's Web site at **http://www.health.gov/NHIC/** or contact an information specialist by calling 1-800-336-4797.

DIRLINE

A comprehensive source of information on associations is the DIRLINE database maintained by the National Library of Medicine. The database comprises some 10,000 records of organizations, research centers, and government institutes and associations which primarily focus on health and biomedicine. DIRLINE is available via the Internet at the following Web site: **http://dirline.nlm.nih.gov/**. Simply type in "aphasia" (or a synonym) or the name of a topic, and the site will list information contained in the database on all relevant organizations.

The Combined Health Information Database

Another comprehensive source of information on healthcare associations is the Combined Health Information Database. Using the "Detailed Search" option, you will need to limit your search to "Organizations" and "aphasia". Type the following hyperlink into your Web browser: **http://chid.nih.gov/detail/detail.html**. To find associations, use the drop boxes at the bottom of the search page where "You may refine your search by." For publication date, select "All Years." Then, select your preferred language and the format option "Organization Resource Sheet." By making these selections and typing in "aphasia" (or synonyms) into the "For these words:" box, you will only receive results on organizations dealing with aphasia. You should check back periodically with this database since it is updated every 3 months.

The National Organization for Rare Disorders, Inc.

The National Organization for Rare Disorders, Inc. has prepared a Web site that provides, at no charge, lists of associations organized by specific diseases. You can access this database at the following Web site: **http://www.rarediseases.org/cgi-bin/nord/searchpage**. Select the option called "Organizational Database (ODB)" and type "aphasia" (or a synonym) in the search box.

Online Support Groups

In addition to support groups, commercial Internet service providers offer forums and chat rooms for people with different illnesses and conditions. WebMD®, for example, offers such a service at their Web site: **http://boards.webmd.com/roundtable**. These online self-help communities can help you connect with a network of people whose concerns are similar to yours. Online support groups are places where people can talk informally. If you read about a novel approach, consult with your doctor or other healthcare providers, as the treatments or discoveries you hear about may not be scientifically proven to be safe and effective.

- **Aphasia Support Group**
  www.indiana.edu/~aphasia

- **NAA: Aphasia Community Groups**
  www.aphasia.org/NAAcommunity.html

- **Mercy Medical Center**
  www.mercycares.com/calendar.asp

Finding Doctors

One of the most important aspects of your treatment will be the relationship between you and your doctor or specialist. All patients with aphasia must go through the process of selecting a physician. While this process will vary from person to person, the Agency for Healthcare Research and Quality makes a number of suggestions, including the following:[10]

- If you are in a managed care plan, check the plan's list of doctors first.

- Ask doctors or other health professionals who work with doctors, such as hospital nurses, for referrals.

- Call a hospital's doctor referral service, but keep in mind that these services usually refer you to doctors on staff at that particular hospital. The services do not have information on the quality of care that these doctors provide.

- Some local medical societies offer lists of member doctors. Again, these lists do not have information on the quality of care that these doctors provide.

Additional steps you can take to locate doctors include the following:

- Check with the associations listed earlier in this chapter.

- Information on doctors in some states is available on the Internet at **http://www.docboard.org**. This Web site is run by "Administrators in Medicine," a group of state medical board directors.

---

[10] This section is adapted from the AHRQ: **www.ahrq.gov/consumer/qntascii/qntdr.htm** .

- The American Board of Medical Specialties can tell you if your doctor is board certified. "Certified" means that the doctor has completed a training program in a specialty and has passed an exam, or "board," to assess his or her knowledge, skills, and experience to provide quality patient care in that specialty. Primary care doctors may also be certified as specialists. The AMBS Web site is located at **http://www.abms.org/newsearch.asp**.[11] You can also contact the ABMS by phone at 1-866-ASK-ABMS.

- You can call the American Medical Association (AMA) at 800-665-2882 for information on training, specialties, and board certification for many licensed doctors in the United States. This information also can be found in "Physician Select" at the AMA's Web site: **http://www.ama-assn.org/aps/amahg.htm**.

Finding an Otolaryngologist

An otolaryngologist is a medical doctor who specializes in the treatment of the ear, nose, throat, and related structures of the head and neck. The American Academy of Otolaryngology—Head and Neck Surgery (AAO-HNS) has created a "Find an Otolaryngologist" searchable database which contains information on the AAO-HNS's 9,300 members. To search the database, go to **http://www.entlink.net/aao-hns_otolaryngologist.cfm**. You will be given the option to search by the following criteria: doctor's name, city, state, zip code, country, or sub-specialty.

If the previous sources did not meet your needs, you may want to log on to the Web site of the National Organization for Rare Disorders (NORD) at **http://www.rarediseases.org/**. NORD maintains a database of doctors with expertise in various rare diseases. The Metabolic Information Network (MIN), 800-945-2188, also maintains a database of physicians with expertise in various metabolic diseases.

---

[11] While board certification is a good measure of a doctor's knowledge, it is possible to receive quality care from doctors who are not board certified.

Selecting Your Doctor[12]

When you have compiled a list of prospective doctors, call each of their offices. First, ask if the doctor accepts your health insurance plan and if he or she is taking new patients. If the doctor is not covered by your plan, ask yourself if you are prepared to pay the extra costs. The next step is to schedule a visit with your chosen physician. During the first visit you will have the opportunity to evaluate your doctor and to find out if you feel comfortable with him or her. Ask yourself, did the doctor:

- Give me a chance to ask questions about aphasia?

- Really listen to my questions?

- Answer in terms I understood?

- Show respect for me?

- Ask me questions?

- Make me feel comfortable?

- Address the health problem(s) I came with?

- Ask me my preferences about different kinds of treatments for aphasia?

- Spend enough time with me?

Trust your instincts when deciding if the doctor is right for you. But remember, it might take time for the relationship to develop. It takes more than one visit for you and your doctor to get to know each other.

Working with Your Doctor[13]

Research has shown that patients who have good relationships with their doctors tend to be more satisfied with their care and have better results. Here are some tips to help you and your doctor become partners:

- You know important things about your symptoms and your health history. Tell your doctor what you think he or she needs to know.

- It is important to tell your doctor personal information, even if it makes you feel embarrassed or uncomfortable.

---

[12] This section has been adapted from the AHRQ: **www.ahrq.gov/consumer/qntascii/qntdr.htm**.
[13] This section has been adapted from the AHRQ: **www.ahrq.gov/consumer/qntascii/qntdr.htm**.

- Bring a "health history" list with you (and keep it up to date).

- Always bring any medications you are currently taking with you to the appointment, or you can bring a list of your medications including dosage and frequency information. Talk about any allergies or reactions you have had to your medications.

- Tell your doctor about any natural or alternative medicines you are taking.

- Bring other medical information, such as x-ray films, test results, and medical records.

- Ask questions. If you don't, your doctor will assume that you understood everything that was said.

- Write down your questions before your visit. List the most important ones first to make sure that they are addressed.

- Consider bringing a friend with you to the appointment to help you ask questions. This person can also help you understand and/or remember the answers.

- Ask your doctor to draw pictures if you think that this would help you understand.

- Take notes. Some doctors do not mind if you bring a tape recorder to help you remember things, but always ask first.

- Let your doctor know if you need more time. If there is not time that day, perhaps you can speak to a nurse or physician assistant on staff or schedule a telephone appointment.

- Take information home. Ask for written instructions. Your doctor may also have brochures and audio and videotapes that can help you.

- After leaving the doctor's office, take responsibility for your care. If you have questions, call. If your symptoms get worse or if you have problems with your medication, call. If you had tests and do not hear from your doctor, call for your test results. If your doctor recommended that you have certain tests, schedule an appointment to get them done. If your doctor said you should see an additional specialist, make an appointment.

By following these steps, you will enhance the relationship you will have with your physician.

Broader Health-Related Resources

In addition to the references above, the NIH has set up guidance Web sites that can help patients find healthcare professionals. These include:[14]

- Caregivers:
  http://www.nlm.nih.gov/medlineplus/caregivers.html

- Choosing a Doctor or Healthcare Service:
  **http://www.nlm.nih.gov/medlineplus/choosingadoctororhealthcareserv
  ice.html**

- Hospitals and Health Facilities:
  http://www.nlm.nih.gov/medlineplus/healthfacilities.html

---

[14] You can access this information at:
http://www.nlm.nih.gov/medlineplus/healthsystem.html.

CHAPTER 3. CLINICAL TRIALS AND APHASIA

Overview

Very few medical conditions have a single treatment. The basic treatment guidelines that your physician has discussed with you, or those that you have found using the techniques discussed in Chapter 1, may provide you with all that you will require. For some patients, current treatments can be enhanced with new or innovative techniques currently under investigation. In this chapter, we will describe how clinical trials work and show you how to keep informed of trials concerning aphasia.

What Is a Clinical Trial?[15]

Clinical trials involve the participation of people in medical research. Most medical research begins with studies in test tubes and on animals. Treatments that show promise in these early studies may then be tried with people. The only sure way to find out whether a new treatment is safe, effective, and better than other treatments for aphasia is to try it on patients in a clinical trial.

---

[15] The discussion in this chapter has been adapted from the NIH and the NEI: **www.nei.nih.gov/netrials/ctivr.htm**.

What Kinds of Clinical Trials Are There?

Clinical trials are carried out in three phases:

- **Phase I.** Researchers first conduct Phase I trials with small numbers of patients and healthy volunteers. If the new treatment is a medication, researchers also try to determine how much of it can be given safely.

- **Phase II.** Researchers conduct Phase II trials in small numbers of patients to find out the effect of a new treatment on aphasia.

- **Phase III.** Finally, researchers conduct Phase III trials to find out how new treatments for aphasia compare with standard treatments already being used. Phase III trials also help to determine if new treatments have any side effects. These trials--which may involve hundreds, perhaps thousands, of people--can also compare new treatments with no treatment.

How Is a Clinical Trial Conducted?

Various organizations support clinical trials at medical centers, hospitals, universities, and doctors' offices across the United States. The "principal investigator" is the researcher in charge of the study at each facility participating in the clinical trial. Most clinical trial researchers are medical doctors, academic researchers, and specialists. The "clinic coordinator" knows all about how the study works and makes all the arrangements for your visits.

All doctors and researchers who take part in the study on aphasia carefully follow a detailed treatment plan called a protocol. This plan fully explains how the doctors will treat you in the study. The "protocol" ensures that all patients are treated in the same way, no matter where they receive care.

Clinical trials are controlled. This means that researchers compare the effects of the new treatment with those of the standard treatment. In some cases, when no standard treatment exists, the new treatment is compared with no treatment. Patients who receive the new treatment are in the treatment group. Patients who receive a standard treatment or no treatment are in the "control" group. In some clinical trials, patients in the treatment group get a new medication while those in the control group get a placebo. A placebo is a harmless substance, a "dummy" pill, that has no effect on aphasia. In other clinical trials, where a new surgery or device (not a medicine) is being tested, patients in the control group may receive a "sham treatment." This treatment, like a placebo, has no effect on aphasia and does not harm patients.

Researchers assign patients "randomly" to the treatment or control group. This is like flipping a coin to decide which patients are in each group. If you choose to participate in a clinical trial, you will not know which group you will be appointed to. The chance of any patient getting the new treatment is about 50 percent. You cannot request to receive the new treatment instead of the placebo or sham treatment. Often, you will not know until the study is over whether you have been in the treatment group or the control group. This is called a "masked" study. In some trials, neither doctors nor patients know who is getting which treatment. This is called a "double masked" study. These types of trials help to ensure that the perceptions of the patients or doctors will not affect the study results.

Natural History Studies

Unlike clinical trials in which patient volunteers may receive new treatments, natural history studies provide important information to researchers on how aphasia develops over time. A natural history study follows patient volunteers to see how factors such as age, sex, race, or family history might make some people more or less at risk for aphasia. A natural history study may also tell researchers if diet, lifestyle, or occupation affects how a disease or disorder develops and progresses. Results from these studies provide information that helps answer questions such as: How fast will a disease or disorder usually progress? How bad will the condition become? Will treatment be needed?

What Is Expected of Patients in a Clinical Trial?

Not everyone can take part in a clinical trial for a specific disease or disorder. Each study enrolls patients with certain features or eligibility criteria. These criteria may include the type and stage of disease or disorder, as well as, the age and previous treatment history of the patient. You or your doctor can contact the sponsoring organization to find out more about specific clinical trials and their eligibility criteria. If you are interested in joining a clinical trial, your doctor must contact one of the trial's investigators and provide details about your diagnosis and medical history.

If you participate in a clinical trial, you may be required to have a number of medical tests. You may also need to take medications and/or undergo surgery. Depending upon the treatment and the examination procedure, you may be required to receive inpatient hospital care. Or, you may have to return to the medical facility for follow-up examinations. These exams help find out how well the treatment is working. Follow-up studies can take months or years. However, the success of the clinical trial often depends on learning what happens to patients over a long period of time. Only patients who continue to return for follow-up examinations can provide this important long-term information.

Recent Trials on Aphasia

The National Institutes of Health and other organizations sponsor trials on various diseases and disorders. Because funding for research goes to the medical areas that show promising research opportunities, it is not possible for the NIH or others to sponsor clinical trials for every disease and disorder at all times. The following lists recent trials dedicated to aphasia.[16] If the trial listed by the NIH is still recruiting, you may be eligible. If it is no longer recruiting or has been completed, then you can contact the sponsors to learn more about the study and, if published, the results. Further information on the trial is available at the Web site indicated. Please note that some trials may no longer be recruiting patients or are otherwise closed. Before contacting sponsors of a clinical trial, consult with your physician who can help you determine if you might benefit from participation.

- **Testing a Possible Cause of Reduced Ability of Children to Process Speech in Noise**

  Condition(s): Central Auditory Disease; Healthy

  Study Status: This study is currently recruiting patients.

  Sponsor(s): National Institute on Deafness and Other Communication Disorders (NIDCD)

  Purpose - Excerpt: This study aims to increase our understanding of the difficulty people have recognizing the spoken word, especially in noisy situations. Subjects must be between 12 and 18 years old with no history of voice disorder, autism, stuttering, aphasia, multiple sclerosis, traumatic brain injury, severe language disorders, and psychiatric disorders. Group A subjects must show reduced speech-in-noise scores and Group B subjects must demonstrate speech-in-noise scores within normal limits. The child will perform a series of hearing tasks that will take from 1.5 to 2 hours, with a break halfway through. A routine hearing test will be given. The child will sit in a sound-treated room wearing

---

[16] These are listed at **www.ClinicalTrials.gov**.

earphones and will depress a button in response to sound or to repeat words. The words may be in quiet or mixed with noise. In a test called "immitance," air pressure change and tones will be sent through a miniature probe in the ear for about 1 minute. TEOAE (transient-evoked otoacoustic emission) testing will test the inner ear with clicking sounds. At times, noise will be presented through a probe in the opposite ear. The child will listen to a series of recordings of speech in quiet and in noise and will be asked to repeat what is heard. These recordings will include monosyllabic words with some part of the sounds cut out; words presented with several voices speaking together; two words presented at the same time, one to each ear (child must repeat both words); and two sentences presented at the same time, one to each ear (child must repeat sentence presented to chosen ear). The only risk in this study is tiredness from listening.

Study Type: Observational

Contact(s): Maryland; National Institute on Deafness and Other Communication Disorders (NIDCD), 9000 Rockville Pike Bethesda, Maryland, 20892, United States; Recruiting; Patient Recruitment and Public Liaison Office 1-800-411-1222 prpl@mail.cc.nih.gov; TTY 1-866-411-1010

Web Site: http://clinicaltrials.gov/ct/gui/c/w2r/show/NCT00001957

- **AERs in Aphasia: Severity and Improvement**

  Condition(s): Stroke

  Study Status: This study is no longer recruiting patients.

  Sponsor(s): Department of Veterans Affairs

  Purpose - Excerpt: Over one million persons in the United States are aphasic subsequent to a stroke. Most of the individuals improve through spontaneous recovery and treatment. However, there are no precise methods for predicting which patients will improve and, for those who do, how much improvement will occur. There is a need to improve prognostic precision in aphasia. The purpose of this investigation is to test the precision of auditory evoked responses (AERs) to provide a prognosis for improvement in aphasia subsequent to a left hemisphere thromboembolic infarct. We hypothesize that the presence, absence, and pattern of the AER responses will predict severity of aphasia and prognosis for improvement. Phonemic, phonologic, semantic, and syntactic language tasks will be used to elicit AERs, including the auditory late response, the mismatch negativity response (MMN), the N400, and the P600.

Phase(s): Phase II

Study Type: Observational

Contact(s): see Web site below

Web Site: http://clinicaltrials.gov/ct/gui/c/w2r/show/NCT00013442

Benefits and Risks[17]

What Are the Benefits of Participating in a Clinical Trial?

If you are interested in a clinical trial, it is important to realize that your participation can bring many benefits to you and society at large:

- A new treatment could be more effective than the current treatment for aphasia. Although only half of the participants in a clinical trial receive the experimental treatment, if the new treatment is proved to be more effective and safer than the current treatment, then those patients who did not receive the new treatment during the clinical trial may be among the first to benefit from it when the study is over.

- If the treatment is effective, then it may improve health or prevent diseases or disorders.

- Clinical trial patients receive the highest quality of medical care. Experts watch them closely during the study and may continue to follow them after the study is over.

- People who take part in trials contribute to scientific discoveries that may help other people with aphasia. In cases where certain diseases or disorders run in families, your participation may lead to better care or prevention for your family members.

The Informed Consent

Once you agree to take part in a clinical trial, you will be asked to sign an "informed consent." This document explains a clinical trial's risks and benefits, the researcher's expectations of you, and your rights as a patient.

---

[17] This section has been adapted from ClinicalTrials.gov, a service of the National Institutes of Health:
http://www.clinicaltrials.gov/ct/gui/c/a1r/info/whatis?JServSessionIdzone_ct=9jmun6f291.

What Are the Risks?

Clinical trials may involve risks as well as benefits. Whether or not a new treatment will work cannot be known ahead of time. There is always a chance that a new treatment may not work better than a standard treatment. There is also the possibility that it may be harmful. The treatment you receive may cause side effects that are serious enough to require medical attention.

How Is Patient Safety Protected?

Clinical trials can raise fears of the unknown. Understanding the safeguards that protect patients can ease some of these fears. Before a clinical trial begins, researchers must get approval from their hospital's Institutional Review Board (IRB), an advisory group that makes sure a clinical trial is designed to protect patient safety. During a clinical trial, doctors will closely watch you to see if the treatment is working and if you are experiencing any side effects. All the results are carefully recorded and reviewed. In many cases, experts from the Data and Safety Monitoring Committee carefully monitor each clinical trial and can recommend that a study be stopped at any time. You will only be asked to take part in a clinical trial as a volunteer giving informed consent.

What Are a Patient's Rights in a Clinical Trial?

If you are eligible for a clinical trial, you will be given information to help you decide whether or not you want to participate. As a patient, you have the right to:

- Information on all known risks and benefits of the treatments in the study.

- Know how the researchers plan to carry out the study, for how long, and where.

- Know what is expected of you.

- Know any costs involved for you or your insurance provider.

- Know before any of your medical or personal information is shared with other researchers involved in the clinical trial.

- Talk openly with doctors and ask any questions.

After you join a clinical trial, you have the right to:

- Leave the study at any time. Participation is strictly voluntary. However, you should not enroll if you do not plan to complete the study.

- Receive any new information about the new treatment.

- Continue to ask questions and get answers.

- Maintain your privacy. Your name will not appear in any reports based on the study.

- Know whether you participated in the treatment group or the control group (once the study has been completed).

What about Costs?

In some clinical trials, the research facility pays for treatment costs and other associated expenses. You or your insurance provider may have to pay for costs that are considered standard care. These things may include inpatient hospital care, laboratory and other tests, and medical procedures. You also may need to pay for travel between your home and the clinic. You should find out about costs before committing to participation in the trial. If you have health insurance, find out exactly what it will cover. If you don't have health insurance, or if your insurance company will not cover your costs, talk to the clinic staff about other options for covering the cost of your care.

What Should You Ask before Deciding to Join a Clinical Trial?

Questions you should ask when thinking about joining a clinical trial include the following:

- What is the purpose of the clinical trial?

- What are the standard treatments for aphasia? Why do researchers think the new treatment may be better? What is likely to happen to me with or without the new treatment?

- What tests and treatments will I need? Will I need surgery? Medication? Hospitalization?

- How long will the treatment last? How often will I have to come back for follow-up exams?

- What are the treatment's possible benefits to my condition? What are the short- and long-term risks? What are the possible side effects?

- Will the treatment be uncomfortable? Will it make me feel sick? If so, for how long?

- How will my health be monitored?

- Where will I need to go for the clinical trial? How will I get there?

- How much will it cost to be in the study? What costs are covered by the study? How much will my health insurance cover?

- Will I be able to see my own doctor? Who will be in charge of my care?

- Will taking part in the study affect my daily life? Do I have time to participate?

- How do I feel about taking part in a clinical trial? Are there family members or friends who may benefit from my contributions to new medical knowledge?

Keeping Current on Clinical Trials

Various government agencies maintain databases on trials. The U.S. National Institutes of Health, through the National Library of Medicine, has developed ClinicalTrials.gov to provide patients, family members, and physicians with current information about clinical research across the broadest number of diseases and conditions.

The site was launched in February 2000 and currently contains approximately 5,700 clinical studies in over 59,000 locations worldwide, with most studies being conducted in the United States. ClinicalTrials.gov receives about 2 million hits per month and hosts approximately 5,400 visitors daily. To access this database, simply go to their Web site (**www.clinicaltrials.gov**) and search by "aphasia" (or synonyms).

While ClinicalTrials.gov is the most comprehensive listing of NIH-supported clinical trials available, not all trials are in the database. The database is updated regularly, so clinical trials are continually being added. The following is a list of specialty databases affiliated with the National Institutes of Health that offer additional information on trials:

- For clinical studies at the Warren Grant Magnuson Clinical Center located in Bethesda, Maryland, visit their Web site: **http://clinicalstudies.info.nih.gov/**

- For clinical studies conducted at the Bayview Campus in Baltimore, Maryland, visit their Web site: **http://www.jhbmc.jhu.edu/studies/index.html**

- For hearing-related trials, visit the National Institute on Deafness and Other Communication Disorders: **http://www.nidcd.nih.gov/health/clinical/index.htm**

General References

The following references describe clinical trials and experimental medical research. They have been selected to ensure that they are likely to be available from your local or online bookseller or university medical library. These references are usually written for healthcare professionals, so you may consider consulting with a librarian or bookseller who might recommend a particular reference. The following includes some of the most readily available references (sorted alphabetically by title; hyperlinks provide rankings, information and reviews at Amazon.com):

- **A Guide to Patient Recruitment : Today's Best Practices & Proven Strategies** by Diana L. Anderson; Paperback - 350 pages (2001), CenterWatch, Inc.; ISBN: 1930624115; **http://www.amazon.com/exec/obidos/ASIN/1930624115/icongroupinterna**

- **A Step-By-Step Guide to Clinical Trials** by Marilyn Mulay, R.N., M.S., OCN; Spiral-bound - 143 pages Spiral edition (2001), Jones & Bartlett Pub; ISBN: 0763715697; **http://www.amazon.com/exec/obidos/ASIN/0763715697/icongroupinterna**

- **The CenterWatch Directory of Drugs in Clinical Trials** by CenterWatch; Paperback - 656 pages (2000), CenterWatch, Inc.; ISBN: 0967302935; **http://www.amazon.com/exec/obidos/ASIN/0967302935/icongroupinterna**

- **The Complete Guide to Informed Consent in Clinical Trials** by Terry Hartnett (Editor); Paperback - 164 pages (2000), PharmSource Information Services, Inc.; ISBN: 0970153309; **http://www.amazon.com/exec/obidos/ASIN/0970153309/icongroupinterna**

- **Dictionary for Clinical Trials** by Simon Day; Paperback - 228 pages (1999), John Wiley & Sons; ISBN: 0471985961; **http://www.amazon.com/exec/obidos/ASIN/0471985961/icongroupinterna**

- **Extending Medicare Reimbursement in Clinical Trials** by Institute of Medicine Staff (Editor), et al; Paperback 1st edition (2000), National Academy Press; ISBN: 0309068886; **http://www.amazon.com/exec/obidos/ASIN/0309068886/icongroupinterna**

- **Handbook of Clinical Trials** by Marcus Flather (Editor); Paperback (2001), Remedica Pub Ltd; ISBN: 1901346293; http://www.amazon.com/exec/obidos/ASIN/1901346293/icongroupinterna

Vocabulary Builder

The following vocabulary builder gives definitions of words used in this chapter that have not been defined in previous chapters:

Auditory: Pertaining to the sense of hearing. [EU]

Tone: 1. the normal degree of vigour and tension; in muscle, the resistance to passive elongation or stretch; tonus. 2. a particular quality of sound or of voice. 3. to make permanent, or to change, the colour of silver stain by chemical treatment, usually with a heavy metal. [EU]

PART II: ADDITIONAL RESOURCES AND ADVANCED MATERIAL

ABOUT PART II

In Part II, we introduce you to additional resources and advanced research on aphasia. All too often, patients who conduct their own research are overwhelmed by the difficulty in finding and organizing information. The purpose of the following chapters is to provide you an organized and structured format to help you find additional information resources on aphasia. In Part II, as in Part I, our objective is not to interpret the latest advances on aphasia or render an opinion. Rather, our goal is to give you access to original research and to increase your awareness of sources you may not have already considered. In this way, you will come across the advanced materials often referred to in pamphlets, books, or other general works. Once again, some of this material is technical in nature, so consultation with a professional familiar with aphasia is suggested.

CHAPTER 4. STUDIES ON APHASIA

Overview

Every year, academic studies are published on aphasia or related conditions. Broadly speaking, there are two types of studies. The first are peer reviewed. Generally, the content of these studies has been reviewed by scientists or physicians. Peer-reviewed studies are typically published in scientific journals and are usually available at medical libraries. The second type of studies is non-peer reviewed. These works include summary articles that do not use or report scientific results. These often appear in the popular press, newsletters, or similar periodicals.

In this chapter, we will show you how to locate peer-reviewed references and studies on aphasia. We will begin by discussing research that has been summarized and is free to view by the public via the Internet. We then show you how to generate a bibliography on aphasia and teach you how to keep current on new studies as they are published or undertaken by the scientific community.

The Combined Health Information Database

The Combined Health Information Database summarizes studies across numerous federal agencies. To limit your investigation to research studies and aphasia, you will need to use the advanced search options. First, go to **http://chid.nih.gov/index.html**. From there, select the "Detailed Search" option (or go directly to that page with the following hyperlink: **http://chid.nih.gov/detail/detail.html**). The trick in extracting studies is found in the drop boxes at the bottom of the search page where "You may refine your search by." Select the dates and language you prefer, and the format option "Journal Article." At the top of the search form, select the number of records you would like to see (we recommend 100) and check the box to display "whole records." We recommend that you type in "aphasia" (or synonyms) into the "For these words:" box. Consider using the option "anywhere in record" to make your search as broad as possible. If you want to limit the search to only a particular field, such as the title of the journal, then select this option in the "Search in these fields" drop box. The following is a sample of what you can expect from this type of search:

- **Consider PCs for Long-Term Aphasia Therapy**

  Source: Advance for Speech-Language Pathologists [and] Audiologists. 6(38): 17. September 23, 1996.

  Summary: This article, from a professional newsletter for speech-language pathologists and audiologists, describes the benefits of home computers for stroke survivors in their search for language retrieval. Benefits are especially great for those who have been discharged from a formal therapy program but have not given up hope of making further gains in recovering language skills. The author proposes a new approach for clients who have been discharged from clinical programs because of lack of progress. Topics include the likelihood of continued progress; addressing the client's need to continue therapy after discharge; the software programs utilized, including language retrieval modules for grammar and spelling and the recording of speech; and recommendations for scheduling home sessions. The article concludes with the address and telephone number of the author.

- **Dementia in the Severely Aphasic: Global Aphasia Without Hemiparesis -- A Stroke Subtype Simulating Dementia**

  Source: American Journal of Alzheimer's Disease. 14(2): 74-78. March-April 1999.

  Summary: This journal article provides case reports of four patients who were referred for evaluation of probable dementia and were found to have severe aphasia over 3 or more years without a history of any other neurological impairment such as hemiplegia. The study examined the utility of several commonly used dementia scales in patients with severe aphasia and possible dementia. Findings identify the limitations of verbal and non-verbal cognitive tests and the reliance on informant reports. Additionally, the authors suggest appropriate weighting of these tests may help in arriving at a more accurate diagnosis; and until guidelines for reliable criteria are established, the clinician should assess the patient in a holistic way rather than in only one aspect of the patient's symptomatology. Data are provided from test results using the Boston

Diagnostic Aphasia Examination at onset, 3 years, and past 3 years. 1 table, 24 references.

- **Development of Aphasia, Apraxia, and Agnosia and Decline in Alzheimer's Disease**

Source: American Journal of Psychiatry. 150(5): 742-747. May 1993.

Summary: This case series study examined whether the rate of clinical decline varied among persons with Alzheimer's disease who showed early development of aphasia (dysfunction in using language), apraxia (dysfunction in ability to carry out actions), and/or agnosia (dysfunction in recognizing what should be familiar). Study participants were administered the Mini-Mental State Examination (MMSE) every 6-12 months; each participant was assessed at least three times. Results showed that participants who developed aphasia and apraxia declined more rapidly on the MMSE than those who did not. These results suggest that Alzheimer's disease does not progress through a series of stages. Rather, they support the notion that there are distinct subtypes of Alzheimer's disease, each of which may have its own pattern of decline. In this case, it seems that accelerated decline is associated with the relatively early onset of certain neurological signs. 22 references.

- **Aphasia Management During the Early Phases of Recovery Following Stroke**

Source: American Journal of Speech-Language Pathology. 10(1): 19-28. February 2001.

Contact: Available from American Speech-Language-Hearing Association (ASHA). Subscription Sales Coordinator, 10801 Rockville Pike, Rockville, MD 20852-3279. (888) 498-6699. Fax (301) 897-7358. Website: www.asha.org.

Summary: Training in speech language pathology seldom distinguishes treatment of aphasia (complete or partial impairment in language comprehension) in its early phases from treatment that occurs when aphasia has become more chronic. This article proposes an approach to therapy for the early phases of recovery following stroke that emphasizes the provision of support, prevention, and education, rather than structured language therapy. The authors first define the period of treatment under discussion, then review the literature in this area. The next section reviews the medical considerations of the newly aphasic patient, and the psychological considerations for both patients and their families. The authors then discuss clinicians' roles with patients in the areas of assessment, the setting of therapy (in the patient's room, generally), early therapy, the conversational approach, the functions of counseling, and aphasia management with families. Other topics include modeling communication strategies for family members, team communication, and reimbursement issues. The authors reiterate that, whenever possible, and to the best of patients', families' and therapists' abilities, positive emotions such as warmth, grace, good humor, and laughter should be sought and cherished in the early aftermath of stroke. 2 tables. 34 references.

- **Supporting Partners of People with Aphasia in Relationships and Conversation (SPPARC)**

Source: International Journal of Language and Communication Disorders. 36(Supplement): 25-30. 2001.

Contact: Available from Taylor and Francis Inc. 1900 Frost Road, Suite 101, Bristol, PA 19007.

Summary: This article reviews new theoretical and practical developments in working with partners of people with aphasia and describes the development of a clinician's resource entitled, 'SPPARC: Supporting Partners of People With Aphasia in Relationships and Conversation.' The authors focus particularly on one part of that resource: the SPPARC Conversation Training Programme, which adapts conversation analysis for clinical use. The authors describe the stages involved in assessing and working on conversation in everyday life. Because conversation is an orderly and finely organized activity, the authors assess and treat the conversation of people with aphasia and their partners not only for what it call tell about language functioning, functional communication or psychosocial issues, but as an activity worthy of attention in its own right. The six steps involved are: preparation, recording the conversation, preliminary viewing of the recording and transcription, conversation assessment, moving from assessment to training, and conversation training. 15 references.

- **Phonological and Orthographic Approaches to the Treatment of Word Retrieval in Aphasia**

Source: International Journal of Language and Communication Disorders. 36(Supplement): 7-12. 2001.

Contact: Available from Taylor and Francis Inc. 1900 Frost Road, Suite 101, Bristol, PA 19007.

Summary: This article presents a preliminary report on a study of the treatment of word finding difficulties in aphasia (a disorder of language comprehension) using phonological and orthographic cues. These techniques, although often used to cue word finding in the immediate term, have seldom been evaluated in terms of therapy designed to improve word retrieval in the long term. The first phase, using cued word retrieval in a picture naming task, was followed by a second phase designed to facilitate use of treated words in real life contexts. The results from both phases were encouraging, with improved word retrieval for three out of the four participants. The authors discuss the implications for clinical practice, noting that generalization effects are particularly encouraging, as they might not be expected in a treatment such as that used here when participants are encouraged to reflect upon an individual word's form (sound or letter) and not to think more widely about words in general. Treatments that can engender a generalized improvement are, however, more beneficial to the individual with aphasia, and are more cost effective in terms of treatment hours. 3 tables. 14 references.

- **Training Volunteers as Conversation Partners Using 'Supported Conversation for Adults with Aphasia' (SCA): A Controlled Trial**

Source: Journal of Speech, Language, and Hearing Research. 44(3): 624-638. June 2001.

Contact: Available from American Speech-Language-Hearing Association (ASHA). Subscription Sales Coordinator, 10801 Rockville Pike, Rockville, MD 20852-3279. (888) 498-6699. Fax (301) 897-7358. Website: www.asha.org.

Summary: This article reports the development and evaluation of a new intervention termed 'Supported Conversation for Adults with Aphasia' (SCA). The approach is based on the idea that the inherent competence of people with aphasia can be revealed through the skills of a conversation partner. The intervention approach was developed at a community based aphasia center where volunteers interact with individuals with chronic aphasia and their families. The experimental study was designed to test whether training improves the conversational skills of volunteers and, if so, whether the improvements affect the communication of their conversation partners with aphasia. Twenty volunteers received SCA training, and 20 control volunteers were merely exposed to people with aphasia. Comparisons between the groups' scores provide support for the efficacy of SCA. Trained volunteers scored significantly higher than untrained volunteers on ratings of acknowledging competence and revealing competence of their partners with aphasia. The training also produced a positive change in ratings of social and message exchange skills of individuals with aphasia, even though these individuals did not participate in the training. The authors discuss the implications of this study for the treatment of aphasia and as an argument for a social model of intervention. 2 appendices. 4 tables. 47 references.

- **Stroke-Associated Stuttering**

Source: Archives of Neurology. 56(5): 624-627. May 1999.

Contact: Available from American Medical Association. Subscriber Services, P.O. Box 10946, Chicago, IL 60610-0946. (800) 262-3250 or (312) 670-7827. Fax (312) 464-5831. E-mail: ama-subs@ama-assn.org. Website: www.ama-assn.org/neuro.

Summary: This article discusses a series of patients whose stuttering speech is associated with stroke. The study was a four case series with follow up for 5 years, or until the stuttering resolved. Four patients are discussed; each developed stuttering speech in association with an acute ischemic stroke. A 68 year old man developed acute stuttering following a large left middle cerebral artery distribution stroke. A 59 year old man who had stuttered as a child began to stutter 2 months after a left temporal lobe infarction, just as his nonfluent aphasia was improving. Another childhood stutterer, a 59 year old, originally left handed, man developed severe but transient stuttering with a right parietal infarction. A 55 year old man with a left occipital infarction had a right hemianopia and an acquired stutter, for which he was anosognosic (unaware it was happening). The authors conclude that the clinical presentation of stroke associated stuttering is variable, as are the locations of the implicated infarctions. 3 figures. 17 references. (AA-M).

- **Qualitative Study of Feedback in Aphasia Treatment**

Source: American Journal of Speech-Language Pathology. 8(3): 218-230. August 1999.

Contact: Available from American Speech-Language-Hearing Association (ASHA). Subscription Sales Coordinator, 10801 Rockville Pike, Rockville, MD 20852-3279. (888) 498-6699. Fax (301) 897-7358. Website: www.asha.org.

Summary: This article reports on a qualitative research study that was completed using ethnographic and conversation analysis methodologies to explore characteristics and functions of feedback in traditional aphasia treatment sessions. The investigators identified and described multiple functions of clinician feedback based on analysis of 15 aphasia treatment sessions. Feedback not only provided general motivation and shaped targeted language behavior, but also assisted in establishing the discourse structure of treatment and in managing important interactional aspects of the exchange (such as the social functions of treatment). For example, liberal use of feedback might be programmed in order to mediate specific responses, or feedback might be sacrificed when practice within more natural conversational discourse is targeted. The authors conclude that understanding the multiple roles of feedback in treatment interactions might help clinicians improve the efficiency and effectiveness of aphasia treatment and assist in training student clinicians. The authors include 18 examples of client and clinician interchanges and describe what they demonstrate. 1 table. 69 references.

- **Emotional Impact of Aphasia**

Source: Seminars in Speech and Language. 20(1): 19-31. 1999.

Contact: Available from Thieme Medical Publishers, Inc. 333 Seventh Avenue, New York, NY 10001. (800) 782-3488. Fax (212) 947-1112. Website: www.thieme.com.

Summary: This article reviews the negative impact of aphasia (impairment of language comprehension) on emotional well being. Depression is the emotional response that has been examined most, and the authors examine the different causes of depression for people with aphasia. They discuss the relationships between recovery and emotional state and the clinical implications of these relationships, then briefly review issues of drug treatment for depression. The authors conclude that the emotional impact of aphasia can have a marked negative impact on recovery, response to rehabilitation, and psychosocial adjustment. The article concludes with a series of self assessment questions. 1 figure. 1 table. 81 references.

- **Quality of Life with Aphasia**

Source: Seminars in Speech and Language. 20(1): 5-17. 1999.

Contact: Available from Thieme Medical Publishers, Inc. 333 Seventh Avenue, New York, NY 10001. (800) 782-3488. Fax (212) 947-1112. Website: www.thieme.com.

Summary: This article considers quality of life (QOL) issues for people with aphasia (impairment of language comprehension). The author first reviews the problems surrounding definition and measurement of QOL. Dimensions of QOL that have been suggested include elements relating to physical problems, the toxicity dimension (of drug therapy and other therapeutic interventions), body image and mobility, communication, and psychological, interpersonal, spiritual, and financial issues. These issues are placed in the context of wider dimensions of satisfaction and life quality related to individuality, culture, and philosophical and time elements. Research on the illness experience is related to QOL. The author reviews research on QOL after stroke and aphasia. Clinical approaches that integrate models of betterment of life quality in aphasia are suggested. The author focuses on notions of coping in the discussion of adjustment and accommodation to life with aphasia. The article concludes with a section of self assessment questions. 36 references.

- **Psychogenic Impact: Reduced Opportunities for Communication Following Aphasia Can Lead to Feelings of Depression**

    Source: ADVANCE for Speech-Language Pathologists and Audiologists. 8(24): 12-14. June 15, 1998.

    Summary: Psychosocial assessments and intervention are often necessary for patients with aphasia because of reduced opportunities for socialization and a change in role that typically follows stroke. This article, from a professional newsletter for audiologists and speech language pathologists, examines how these reduced opportunities for communication following aphasia can lead to feelings of depression. The article considers several techniques that exist for measuring the psychosocial adjustment of a person with aphasia. The article then describes the programs available through the Aphasia Center at North York, Ontario, Canada. The article also discusses aphasia therapy and its four typical stages: acute, intensive, maintenance, and adaptation. The adaptation phase of rehabilitation is particularly appropriate for intervention related to psychosocial issues because as therapy ends, the family must confront the fact that the patient has reduced opportunities to participate in social and community life. The article concludes with the contact information for the clinicians interviewed, as well as the phone number of the National Aphasia Association (800-922-4622).

- **Crossed Aphasia**

    Source: ADVANCE for Speech-Language Pathologists and Audiologists. 8(24): 7-9. June 15, 1998.

    Summary: This article, from a professional newsletter for audiologists and speech language pathologists, discusses aphasia resulting from a right hemisphere lesion. Most people depend on the left hemisphere of the brain for language, but a right-hemisphere lesion can cause aphasia. Crossed aphasia is a rare syndrome in which a right hemisphere cerebrovascular accident (stroke) in a right handed person causes speaking and writing difficulty; this type occurs in about 5 percent of all people with aphasia. The author presents a case report of crossed aphasia in which a two-month course of speech and language therapy remediated deficits in auditory comprehension, verbal and written expression, reading comprehension, and overall speech pattern. This case report is used as an example to discuss other topics including the neurolinguistic characteristics of crossed aphasia, the prognosis for crossed aphasia, goals for speech language therapy with these patients, reading comprehension, and written expression. The article concludes with the contact information for the clinician interviewed.

- **Treatment of Aphasia**

  Source: Archives of Neurology. 55(11): 1417-1419. November 1998.

  Contact: Available from American Medical Association. Subscriber Services, P.O. Box 10946, Chicago, IL 60610-0946. (800) 262-3250 or (312) 670-7827. Fax (312) 464-5831. E-mail: ama-subs@ama-assn.org. Website: www.ama-assn.org/neuro.

  Summary: Approximately one million people have aphasia in the U.S. today, yet with properly targeted therapy in selected patients, effective communication can be restored. This review article addresses three issues: the relevance of aphasia therapy to neurologists, the current state of the art, and future trends. Linguistic and nonlinguistic cognitive functions, such as attention, memory, and executive system functions, are interdependent and may be affected to different degrees in patients with aphasia. Knowledge of how language can be influenced by nonlinguistic cognitive functions (traditionally assigned to the right hemisphere or considered to be linked to frontosubcortical systems) has been useful in developing new approaches to the treatment of aphasia. The author reviews current approaches to the treatment of aphasia, including psycholinguistic theory driven therapy, cognitive neurorehabilitation, computer aided techniques, psychosocial management, and (still on an experimental basis) pharmacotherapy. 27 references. (AA-M).

- **Treatment Efficacy: Aphasia**

  Source: Journal of Speech and Hearing Research (JSHR). 39(5): S27-S36. October 1996.

  Summary: This article presents a brief overview of aphasia, followed by a summary of research studies and program evaluation data that supports the efficacy of treatment for aphasia. Selected studies are reviewed in terms of the quality of evidence they present. In addition, the authors discuss a number of questions in this area that remain unanswered. Several tables are included, listing several aspects of research design, including number and types of patients studied, examples of well-designed small-group or single-subject studies, and clinical techniques for which efficacy data are available. The authors conclude that generally, treatment for aphasia is efficacious. 4 tables. 60 references. (AA-M).

Federally-Funded Research on Aphasia

The U.S. Government supports a variety of research studies relating to aphasia and associated conditions. These studies are tracked by the Office of Extramural Research at the National Institutes of Health.[18] CRISP (Computerized Retrieval of Information on Scientific Projects) is a searchable database of federally-funded biomedical research projects conducted at universities, hospitals, and other institutions. Visit the CRISP Web site at **http://commons.cit.nih.gov/crisp3/CRISP.Generate_Ticket**. You can perform targeted searches by various criteria including geography, date, as well as topics related to aphasia and related conditions.

For most of the studies, the agencies reporting into CRISP provide summaries or abstracts. As opposed to clinical trial research using patients, many federally-funded studies use animals or simulated models to explore aphasia and related conditions. In some cases, therefore, it may be difficult to understand how some basic or fundamental research could eventually translate into medical practice. The following sample is typical of the type of information found when searching the CRISP database for aphasia:

- **Project Title: Boston University Aphasia Research Core Center**

  Principal Investigator & Institution: Albert, Martin L.; Professor; Neurology; Boston University 121 Bay State Rd Boston, Ma 02215

  Timing: Fiscal Year 2001; Project Start 6-SEP-2001; Project End 1-AUG-2006

  Summary: (provided by applicant): The principal objectives of the Aphasia Research Core Center are to recruit research participants and to provide clinical assessment and data management and analysis services for research projects that advance the theoretical understanding, clinical evaluation, and treatment of language disorders produced by injury or dysfunction of the brain in adults. The Aphasia Research Core Center consists of two cores: a Clinical Assessment Core and a Data Management and Analysis (DAMA) Core, together with administrative support for these cores. The Clinical Assessment Core recruits research participants, provides comprehensive assessments of aphasic, right brain damaged, and healthy elderly subjects, and coordinates their participation in all research projects associated with the Core Center.

---

[18] Healthcare projects are funded by the National Institutes of Health (NIH), Substance Abuse and Mental Health Services (SAMHSA), Health Resources and Services Administration (HRSA), Food and Drug Administration (FDA), Centers for Disease Control and Prevention (CDCP), Agency for Healthcare Research and Quality (AHRQ), and Office of Assistant Secretary of Health (OASH).

Assessment Core examinations include four major components: a medical/neurological evaluation by a behavioral neurologist, a language evaluation, a neuropsychological evaluation, and a neuroimaging evaluation. The Data Management and Analysis Core provides a comprehensive database of all assessment and research data for each research participant. The primary objectives of this core are to manage the data obtained by members of the Clinical Assessment Core and all research projects, to make the data accessible to all ARC researchers, and to provide research design and statistical support for on-going analysis of data and development of new research protocols. The DAMA core has three major service areas: data management, research design and statistical analysis, and education of research investigators. To achieve the overall goals of the Core Center, we intend to support research on language and aphasia within different, but interrelated, disciplines simultaneously. The unifying agenda of the Core Center will be to integrate these various approaches to arrive at a coherent picture of how language is represented in the brain.

Website: http://commons.cit.nih.gov/crisp3/CRISP.Generate_Ticket

- **Project Title: Cross Linguistic Studies in Aphasia**

Principal Investigator & Institution: Bates, Elizabeth A.; Professor; Ctr for Research in Language; University of California San Diego Gilman & La Jolla Village Dr San Diego, Ca 92093

Timing: Fiscal Year 2000; Project Start 1-JUN-1983; Project End 1-JUL-2001

Summary: (Adapted from the Investigator's Abstract): In the proposed research on aphasia, crosslinguistic comparisons allow disentanglement of a confounding between universal mechanisms and language-specific content. New studies are proposed of aphasic patients with lexical and/or grammatical symptoms across languages that differ in lexical and grammatical structure. Experiments are motivated by six findings of the research program over the last 12 years. 1) The same aphasic syndromes look very different from one language to another. This leads the principal investigator and colleagues to propose to compare languages that maximize linguistic contrasts of interest. The languages under study will be Chinese, English, Italian, Spanish and Russian. 2) Language-specific knowledge is largely intact in aphasic patients suggesting that the deficits are in the processes by which knowledge is accessed in real time. That is, deficits are in performance rather than in competence. This account is tested by expanded use of real-time experimental procedures that yield information about how patients arrive at a correct or incorrect response in comprehension and production. 3) Despite these cross-language differences, grammatical inflections and function words are especially vulnerable in every language. This leads to experiments that compare aspects of language that are either at risk or protected within and across language types. 4) Some aspects of grammatical vulnerability show up in every patient group. This finding leads to experiments that assess the contribution of global forms of stress (e.g., perceptual degradation and/or cognitive loads) to isolate those impairments that are specific to particular types of aphasia from those that can be induced in normals under stressed conditions. 5) Despite quantitative differences in vulnerability, the grammatical symptoms displayed by fluent and nonfluent patients are qualitatively similar to their lexical symptoms. This leads to experiments comparing the effects of lexical and grammatical context in languages that rely to different degrees on word order, inflections and/or lexical contrasts to accomplish the same communicative goals. 6) There may be 'neurolinguistic universals'--that is, contrasts among patient groups that are invariant across different language types--that will be investigated. This includes dissociations between nouns and verbs and between closed-class and content words. The proposed studies will help to move the field of aphasiology toward a new model of brain organization for language, integrating universal and language-specific symptoms. The studies also have practical significance for international communication about aphasia, for the development of test batteries for aphasics that are tailored to the specific characteristics of individual languages and for clinical services to the bilingual communities of the nation.

Website: http://commons.cit.nih.gov/crisp3/CRISP.Generate_Ticket

- **Project Title: C-Speak Aphasia Alternative Communication Treatment**

Principal Investigator & Institution: Nicholas, Marjorie L.; Neurology; Boston University 121 Bay State Rd Boston, Ma 02215

Timing: Fiscal Year 2001; Project Start 1-SEP-2001; Project End 1-AUG-2004

Summary: (provided by applicant): This study investigates communicative performance in people with severe restriction in verbal output due to non- fluent aphasia. Such individuals are trained to use an alternative communication program called C-Speak Aphasia. This program is picture-based and operated on a Mackintosh computer. Using C-Speak, patients learn to select icons from semantic-category groups and combine them to form novel messages that can be spoken aloud by the computer s speech synthesizer. This project proposes to conduct a controlled study of treatment outcomes in people with aphasia who are trained to use C-Speak. The study uses a multiple baseline design to determine whether patients improve communication on several tasks while using C-Speak, compared to communication without C-Speak. Communication performance is probed repeatedly during a 46 month training period with 5 tasks; providing autobiographical information, describing pictures and observed events, communicating via writing, and telephone communication. Linguistic factors related to semantic processing and cognitive factors related to executive functioning are hypothesized to be related to individual aphasic patients abilities to communicate using C-Speak. These factors will be assessed during baseline testing, and used as predictors in a multiple regression analysis to investigate whether they predict changes in participants ability to use C- Speak for functional communication. Finally, two experiments relating to semantic functioning and executive system function will also be completed using the subjects who undergo C-Speak training. Scores on these measures will also be used as predictors of successful C-Speak usage.

Website: http://commons.cit.nih.gov/crisp3/CRISP.Generate_Ticket

- **Project Title: Lexical Segmentation and Access in Aphasia**

Principal Investigator & Institution: Gow, David W.; Assistant in Psychology; Massachusetts General Hospital 55 Fruit St Boston, Ma 02114

Timing: Fiscal Year 2000; Project Start 1-FEB-1998; Project End 1-JAN-2003

Summary: (Adapted from the Investigator's Abstract): The long-term goal of this project is to examine lexical segmentation in aphasia, and to use the resulting data to help understand how humans accomplish the difficult task of recognizing individual words in connected speech. The strategy behind the research is to identify patients with specific impairments in targeted aspects of language processing including lexical access, and the discrimination of putative acoustic-phonetic word boundary cues, and examine how they interpret speech sequences known as oronyms in which positing different word boundaries leads to recognizing different words (e.g., kidnap/kid nap). It will address four issues: (1) whether lexical segmentation is the results of a discrete process, or a byproduct of lexical access, (2) how the acoustic form of word onsets affects lexical segmentation, (3) what the timecourse of segmentation disambiguation is, and (4) what factors modulate interword competition in lexical access and/or segmentation. These issues will be examined through a series of offline discrimination tasks and online paradigms including cross-modal lexical priming and word monitoring that provide implicit measures of aphasic and unimpaired listeners' interpretation of oronyms. This research will provide both individual and group studies of lexical access and segmentation and their impairment. At present there are no published studies examining lexical segmentation in aphasia. As segmentation is one of the central problems of spoken word recognition in connected speech processing, this work addresses a critical gap in our understanding of aphasic disturbances of spoken language comprehension. In addition to characterizing the nature of segmentation processes in aphasia, this work will provide a new source of converging evidence to understand the organization of spoken word recognition processes in normal listeners. It is expected that the understanding gained will ultimately be useful to clinicians, therapists and theorists.

Website: http://commons.cit.nih.gov/crisp3/CRISP.Generate_Ticket

- **Project Title: Long Term Aphasia Rehabilitation; Groups, Email, Assisted Communication**

Principal Investigator & Institution: Schwartz, Myrna F.; Associate Director; Moss Rehabilitation Hospital 1200 W Tabor Rd Philadelphia, Pa 19141

Timing: Fiscal Year 2000; Project Start 8-SEP-2000; Project End 0-JUN-2005

Summary: This scientific-project explores how functional communication and quality of life in persons with aphasia are affected by having the opportunity to form social bonds through communication groups, e-mail, and an innovative, PC-based augmentative communication system (CS). CS functions as a "processing prosthesis," enabling the aphasic speakers to construct messages piecemeal and retain elements already produced. Modifications now underway will add an e-mail component to CS (which we call c-mail) so that the vocal messages constructed with CS can be sent electronically over the Internet. The primary aim of this project is to test this global hypothesis: Hypothesis #1: The combination of supported conversation groups, Internet communication, and CS have a positive effect on language performance, functional communication, and psychological well-being in persons with aphasia. The secondary aim is to fractionate the anticipated positive outcome and evaluate the relative merits of the components of this three-pronged intervention. The following are our hypotheses: Hypotheses #2: Having the opportunity simply to participate in supported conservation groups and e-mail communication (i.e., without CS+C-mail) will itself have a measurable impact on aphasics' language use, functional communication, and/or perceived quality of life. Hypotheses #3: Introducing CS and c-mail in a subsequent phase of the study (Phase 2) will promote incremental gains. Hypothesis #4: The efficacy if CS + c-mail does not require that it be preceded by a lengthy period of conventional e-mail use. Patients who experience CS + c-mail in Phase ` will also show gains in the language, communication, and well-being measures. Hypothesis #5: Subjects will express preference for c-mail over conventional text- or voice e-mail; and when given the opportunity to choose, will elect to use c-mail.

Website: http://commons.cit.nih.gov/crisp3/CRISP.Generate_Ticket

- **Project Title: Microstructure of Verbal Retrieval Failure in Aphasia**

Principal Investigator & Institution: Lindfield, Kimberly C.; Neurology; Boston University 121 Bay State Rd Boston, Ma 02215

Timing: Fiscal Year 2000; Project Start 1-AUG-1999; Project End 0-APR-2002

Summary: The overall goal of the proposed research is to reveal the underlying microstructure of verbal memory retrieval deficits in aphasia through a detailed analysis of the temporal output pattern of free-recall responses in early and later stages of learning. The ability to acquire and retrieve new information is essential to all other aspects of behavior and a better understanding of the mechanisms underlying the breakdowns in aphasia would have particular relevance with regard to aphasia therapy and recovery from aphasia. Five experiments are proposed that are designed to investigate systematically the contributions of organizational and semantic factors to aphasic retrieval deficits. Emphasis will be placed on the contributions of these factors to retrieval deficits in anterior versus posterior aphasic syndromes. Identification of the components of the retrieval failures that are specifically related to language disturbances associated with anterior and posterior aphasic syndromes should be possible from a detailed analysis of the temporal dynamics of free-recall. The research question of particular interest is the extent to which (1) retrieval dynamics of aphasic patients with anterior lesions may be associated with deficits in organizational abilities (executive systems) and (2) the retrieval patterns associated with posterior aphasic patients will be associated with deficits of semantic systems. All experiments will include four subject groups; anterior aphasics, posterior aphasics, left-hemisphere damaged non-aphasic patients, and age-matched normal controls. Participants will be presented with study lists consisting of objects or words that can either be organized into different semantic categories or are unrelated. Study lists will be presented to each subject over multiple successive trials with free-recall following each one. Following the completion of the learning and recall trials, retention of the list items will also be assessed using a recognition format.

Website: http://commons.cit.nih.gov/crisp3/CRISP.Generate_Ticket

- **Project Title: Pharmacologic Modulation in the Treatment of Aphasia**

  Principal Investigator & Institution: Walker-Batson, Delaina; Communication Scis & Disorders; Texas Woman's University Box 22965, Twu Station Denton, Tx 76204

  Timing: Fiscal Year 1998; Project Start 0-SEP-1996; Project End 0-APR-2003

  Summary: (Adapted From The Investigator s Abstract): The long-term goal of this research is to determine the efficacy of pharmacologic modulation in the treatment of aphasia subsequent to stroke with oral doses of d-amphetamine (AMP). This is a double-blind parallel study of the use of AMP to modify or promote recovery from aphasia. This work is a critical extension of a large body of animal studies which have provided strong evidence related to the role of norepinephrine (NE) in central nervous system recover processes. The specific aims of the project are: (1) to determine the efficacy of using pharmacologic modulation in the treatment of aphasia following an occlusive left hemisphere stroke and (2) to provide evaluation of the drug treatment within a double-blind parallel design through a six- week drug treatment period and long-term follow-up. Efficacy will be evaluated by Overall Percentile Scores on the Porch Index of Communicative Abilities. Thirty-two patients will be studied over the three-year course of this study and receive either AMP or placebo over ten alternating treatment sessions and then be followed over 12 months. Additionally, patients will be described neurologically (NIH Stroke Scale) and radiologically (MRI) to further enhance understanding of possible relationships between response/nonresponse to drug therapy. The American Speech and Hearing Association Functional Assessment of Communication Skills (ASHA FACS) will be administered to assess functional communication. The debilitating effects of stroke and aphasia are long-term and represent a major adult health problem. To date, there has been no systematic pharmacologic therapy employed in rehabilitation of aphasia. If a relatively simple pharmacologic treatment with an established drug would be found to accelerate rate and/or extent of recovery from aphasia, it would have wide-reaching application.

  Website: http://commons.cit.nih.gov/crisp3/CRISP.Generate_Ticket

- **Project Title: Relation Between Attention and Language in Aphasia**

  Principal Investigator & Institution: Murray, Laura L.; Speech and Hearing Sciences; Indiana University Bloomington Bryan Hall Bloomington, in 47405

Timing: Fiscal Year 2000; Project Start 1-AUG-1999; Project End 1-JUL-2004

Summary: The proposed research consists of two projects designed to examine the relation between attention and language in adults with aphasia. The working hypothesis is that aphasic adults present with deficits of attentional capacity and allocation, and that these deficits negatively interact with their comprehension and production of spoken language. The purpose of Project 1 is to determine the effects of varying attentional demands (e.g., focused attention vs. divided attention conditions) on the auditory comprehension and spoken language skills of aphasic adults, and to compare these effects to those observed in the performances of adults with no brain-damage. Subjects presenting with a variety of aphasia types and severities will participate to investigate the relation between different language profiles and attentional abilities. The purpose of Project 2 is to delineate the nature of attentional deficits in aphasia; that is, to determine whether impairments of attentional capacity, its allocation, or both underlie the attention deficits of adults with aphasia. On a theoretical basis, the findings from the proposed research will inform models of aphasia, attention, and language. Clinically, this research will contribute to more timely and effective assessment and treatment of aphasia by identifying language symptoms which are more likely to reflect underlying attention as oposed to purely linguistic deficits.

Website: http://commons.cit.nih.gov/crisp3/CRISP.Generate_Ticket

- **Project Title: Sentence Production in Aphasia**

  Principal Investigator & Institution: Caplan, David; Boston University 121 Bay State Rd Boston, Ma 02215

  Timing: Fiscal Year 2000

  Summary: The goal of this project is to investigate the effects of lexical and syntactic factors in sentence production in aphasia. Lexical factors will be divided into those associated with nouns (noun-related semantics), and those associated with verbs (verb argument structure). Syntactic effects to be explored are those associated with word orders that place the agent/actor of a verb before or after the verb (constituent order). The role that these factors play in determining sentence production will be examined for normal subjects and aphasic patients, using a series of different tasks designed to provide converging evidence regarding aphasic patients' performances. These factors will be used as independent variables in experiments in which the ability to produce lexical items, grammatical elements, syntactic structures, and thematic roles will be the dependent measures. The research is designed to provide basic data regarding sentence production in aphasia that is not presently available. These data will related to models of normal sentence production. They may ultimately be useful in guiding therapy directed at improving aphasic patients' sentence production abilities.

Website: http://commons.cit.nih.gov/crisp3/CRISP.Generate_Ticket

- **Project Title: Stimulating Cognitive Processes to Remediate Aphasia**

Principal Investigator & Institution: Holland, Audrey L.; University of Arizona Tucson, Az 85721

Timing: Fiscal Year 2000

Summary: The research proposed here is a series of clinical studies of therapy for individuals with aphasia, directed at the interface between cognitive and linguistic processing. The objective of this research is to provided tested alternatives to traditional aphasia therapy that attempt to modify language performance by direct work on patient deficits. The research has two phases. In Phase I, two groups of studies will use single-case research methods to develop and test a series of innovative cognitively based interventions. One set of these interventions will focus on patients whose aphasia is accompanied by nonverbal cognitive disorders and is directed to remediation for them. The second set of studies in Phase I, will focus on a different set of individuals with aphasia, those who demonstrate good cognitive skills. These studies are aimed at enlisting these good cognitive skills to aid in the development of compensatory support for poor language performance. In Phase II, a group study is proposed. Individuals with aphasia whose cognitive skills are similar to those studied in Phase I, will be tested with the treatments validated in Phase I and their performance will be compared with a matched group of patients treated with direct intervention for their language disorders. In both phases of this project, external criterial tests of cognition, language, and functional language skills will be used to measure comparative effectiveness of the training protocols. All treatment in this study will be provided at an intensity that approximates that of current reimbursed clinical practice, so its usefulness for ongoing clinical environments can be evaluated.

Website: http://commons.cit.nih.gov/crisp3/CRISP.Generate_Ticket

- **Project Title: Syntactic Deficits in Aphasia**

Principal Investigator & Institution: Berndt, Rita S.; Professor; Neurology; University of Maryland Balt Prof School Professional Schools Baltimore, Md 21201

Timing: Fiscal Year 2000; Project Start 1-DEC-1983; Project End 1-DEC-2001

Summary: (Adapted from the Investigator's Abstract): Language disorders resulting from focal brain damage can take a variety of forms, and there is evidence that some aphasic deficits selectively affect the comprehension and interpretation of sentences. This project investigates the functional bases of the sentence processing disorders that occur in aphasia. The specific aims for the next project period involve continued investigation of the contribution of impairments of lexical/semantic representations and/or processes to symptoms involving sentence production and comprehension. Aphasic patients and normal control subjects will participate in a variety of different types of experiments: (1) The contribution of various types of information to lexical retrieval in sentence production will be investigated using tasks combining semantic, syntactic, visual/pictorial, or phonological cues to trigger word retrieval in timed production tasks. These studies will evaluate the relative contribution of these information sources to retrieval of nouns and verbs that are high and low in imageability, and will assess the degree to which competing responses interfere with retrieval. (2) New techniques will be designed to elicit sentences of different structural types from patients by exploiting the factors believed to affect lexical and structural decisions in normal sentence production; the relative effectiveness of these factors will be assessed in a separate set of experiments. (3) The contribution of semantic factors to impairment in the comprehension of reversible sentences will be studied using standard sentence/picture matching and speeded verification. The consequences of verb meanings for thematic role assignment are hypothesized to have specific and measurable effects on patients' comprehension performance. (4) Patients' sensitivity to violations of sentence meaning that are caused by illegal combinations of lexical semantic and structural information will be evaluated using the word monitoring task. Sentence complexity (passive v. active) is expected to attenuate violation detection for patients with poor sentence comprehension. The long-term goal is to develop a model sentence comprehension and production that can provide a functional explanation for the symptoms found in aphasia. Such a model would have a variety of applications. If specific aphasic symptoms can be interpreted as arising from identifiable processing deficits within a testable model, then attempts to remediate symptoms can be more definitely focused on the responsible representation or process. Moreover, discrete components of language processing that are identified through studies of aphasic patients are likely to be the components that will, ultimately, prove to be localizable in the brain.

Website: http://commons.cit.nih.gov/crisp3/CRISP.Generate_Ticket

- **Project Title: Treatment of Aphasia and Related Disorders**

Principal Investigator & Institution: Gonzalez-Rothi, Leslie J.; Neurology; University of Florida Gainesville, Fl 32611

Timing: Fiscal Year 2000; Project Start 1-JUN-2000; Project End 1-MAY-2004

Summary: The mission of the proposed Program Project shall be to foster excellence in research focusing on the rehabilitation of language and related disorders resulting from acquired brain impairment. The Program Project contains four Subprojects and two Core Units. The four Subprojects are designed to develop and study the efficacy of theoretically motivated, behavioral treatments for specified cognitive deficits associated with aphasia using multiple replications of within subject, experimental design, experimental designs. The cognitive deficits targeted for study include agrammatisms, anomia, aprosodia, and attention disorders associated with aphasia. In addition, it is our interest to embed this research into biological underpinnings in two ways. First, predictions about the efficacy of choices of treatment strategy (restitutive versus vicariative/substitutive) in a portion of the Subprojects involve an interpretation at the cellular level of the physiology of the recovering system at different points in the recovery process (acute versus chronic). Second, we plan to study the nature of biological changes in the processing system that result from these experimental behavioral interventions by studying a portion of the experimental subjects using pre- and post-treatment fMRI. Finally, the impact that these behavioral treatment may have on the quality of the lives of participants (including their caregivers) will be monitored via a variety of methods.

Website: http://commons.cit.nih.gov/crisp3/CRISP.Generate_Ticket

- **Project Title: Word Retrieval in Aphasia**

Principal Investigator & Institution: Wingfield, Arthur; Professor; Neurology; Boston University 121 Bay State Rd Boston, Ma 02215

Timing: Fiscal Year 2002; Project Start 1-MAR-2002; Project End 8-FEB-2007

Summary: (provided by applicant): The focus of this research is the study of the brain mechanisms in word retrieval in normal speakers as revealed by their disruption in aphasia, where these mechanisms have become damaged or dissociated. Following an examination of perceptual competition on naming objects in fluent and nonfluent aphasia, the first of a series of experiments addresses the problem of dissociation of noun and verb impairments in Broca's aphasia by adopting Luria's distinction between predicative and nominal modes of speech. The possibility is investigated that this distinction may underlie this commonly observed dissociation. The next stage of this investigation examines the role of semantic memory in word retrieval by examining patients' competence in identifying the properties of objects to be named and comparing this ability with their success in retrieving the names of these objects. The third question in the research focuses on the stages of phonological activation and implementation in word production. A model is proposed to identify the multi-staged nature of phonological activation. Predicted differences in speed of naming following from immediate versus delayed priming of picture names will be tested with the goal of distinguishing between the effects of early and late stages of phonological activation. Finally, a series of three studies using the "gating" technique examines the differences between Broca's and Wernicke's aphasics by comparing their response to priming with word onsets and with the prosody (stress pattern and duration) of target words. This research program promises clinical insights that will be useful in the differential diagnosis of aphasia as well as making theoretical contributions to understanding the mechanisms of word production and phonological realization.

Website: http://commons.cit.nih.gov/crisp3/CRISP.Generate_Ticket

- **Project Title: Contrasting Treatment for Word Retrieval Impairments**

Principal Investigator & Institution: Raymer, Anastasia; University of Florida Gainesville, Fl 32611

Timing: Fiscal Year 2000; Project Start 1-JUN-2000; Project End 1-MAY-2001

Summary: A prominent symptom seen in individuals with aphasia due to left cerebral hemisphere disease is difficulty with word retrieval affecting either nouns or verbs. Recent investigation of treatments for word retrieval impairments have been influenced by cognitive neuropsychological models which recognize that word retrieval involves a complex set of lexical processes including semantic and phonologic stages. Subsequently, studies have incorporated restitutive semantic or phonologic treatments and have demonstrative improvements in word retrieval abilities in some individuals, particularly for nouns. Less attention has been given to examining the effects of substitutive word retrieval treatments that might invoke other cognitive processes, no treatment effects for verbs, and to comparing different treatments in the same individuals with aphasia. In our studies, we propose to develop normative data for a battery of lexical tasks assessing comprehension and production of nouns and verbs. We will later administer the battery the battery to patients with aphasia to document the nature of the word retrieval impairments. We then will complete a series of studies in which we contrast two word retrieval treatments. The restitutive treatment will encourage the use of typical semantic and phonologic word retrieval processes, whereas the substitutive verbal+ gestural treatment will encourage the use of pantomimes to evoke a corresponding verbal response. We will compare treatment effects for both nouns and verbs. We will assess performance in structural word retrieval tasks as well as in conversational and functional measures of treatment outcome. In a final experiment, we will study the neural correlates of treatment effects using fMRI.

Website: http://commons.cit.nih.gov/crisp3/CRISP.Generate_Ticket

- **Project Title: Disorders of Lexical Access in Speech Production**

  Principal Investigator & Institution: Caramazza, Alfonso; Professor; Psychology; Harvard University 1350 Massachusetts Ave, Rm 458 Cambridge, Ma 02138

  Timing: Fiscal Year 2000; Project Start 1-SEP-2000; Project End 1-AUG-2005

  Summary: The goal of the proposed research is to understand the nature of naming and word-finding difficulties in aphasia. The objective is to explain patterns of word production deficits in terms of damage to the cognitive/linguistic mechanisms that underlie normal word production, and then to use this knowledge toward the development of a theory of the functional organization of the brain. Two general questions will be addressed: 1) What are the causes of the grammatical class deficits? And, 2) what are the causes of the different error types in naming deficits? More specific questions include: 1) Are there different subtypes of grammatical class disorders? 2) What is the relationship between impairments in the production of nouns and the ability to produce noun phrase structure? 3) Are the causes of access failure for nouns and verbs the same as for failure to retrieve adjectives? What are the causes of failure to access function words and inflectional morphology? 4) Are different mixtures of error types the result of global lesions that affect equally all stages of the lexical access process or are they the result (at least in some cases) of different lesions to different stages of the process? 5) What relationship is there between the distribution of error types in naming and other tasks (such as reading, repetition, comprehension, etc.)? These and related questions will be addressed through a three-pronged program of research. The most important part involves the detailed investigation of the word and phrase processing performance of English and Italian monolingual aphasics and Spanish-Catalan bilingual aphasics. The two other components of the research involve the computational modeling of the patients' patterns of word production deficits and the experimental investigation of normal subjects' word and phrase production performance. This integrated approach to the study of lexical access deficits should provide important information about the organization and processing structure of the lexicon and about the functional causes of word production disorders in aphasia. These are necessary components of the larger goal of understanding the functional architecture of the brain and for developing intervention strategies for remedial training of aphasia.

Website: http://commons.cit.nih.gov/crisp3/CRISP.Generate_Ticket

E-Journals: PubMed Central[19]

PubMed Central (PMC) is a digital archive of life sciences journal literature developed and managed by the National Center for Biotechnology Information (NCBI) at the U.S. National Library of Medicine (NLM).[20] Access to this growing archive of e-journals is free and unrestricted.[21] To search, go to **http://www.pubmedcentral.nih.gov/index.html#search**, and type "aphasia" (or synonyms) into the search box. This search gives you access to full-text articles. The following is a sample of items found for aphasia in the PubMed Central database:

- **A syntactic specialization for Broca's area** by David Embick, Alec Marantz, Yasushi Miyashita, Wayne O'Neil, and Kuniyoshi L. Sakai; 2000 May 23
  http://www.pubmedcentral.nih.gov/articlerender.fcgi?artid=18573

- **Nouns and Verbs are Retrieved with Differently Distributed Neural Systems** by AR Damasio and D Tranel; 1993 June 1
  http://www.pubmedcentral.nih.gov/articlerender.fcgi?rendertype=abstract&artid=46632

---

[19] Adapted from the National Library of Medicine: **http://www.pubmedcentral.nih.gov/about/intro.html**.

[20] With PubMed Central, NCBI is taking the lead in preservation and maintenance of open access to electronic literature, just as NLM has done for decades with printed biomedical literature. PubMed Central aims to become a world-class library of the digital age.

[21] The value of PubMed Central, in addition to its role as an archive, lies the availability of data from diverse sources stored in a common format in a single repository. Many journals already have online publishing operations, and there is a growing tendency to publish material online only, to the exclusion of print.

- **Preserved Speech Abilities and Compensation Following Prefrontal Damage** by RL Buckner, M Corbetta, J Schatz, ME Raichle, and SE Petersen; 1996 February 6
  http://www.pubmedcentral.nih.gov/articlerender.fcgi?rendertype=abstract&artid=40065

The National Library of Medicine: PubMed

One of the quickest and most comprehensive ways to find academic studies in both English and other languages is to use PubMed, maintained by the National Library of Medicine. The advantage of PubMed over previously mentioned sources is that it covers a greater number of domestic and foreign references. It is also free to the public.[22] If the publisher has a Web site that offers full text of its journals, PubMed will provide links to that site, as well as to sites offering other related data. User registration, a subscription fee, or some other type of fee may be required to access the full text of articles in some journals.

To generate your own bibliography of studies dealing with aphasia, simply go to the PubMed Web site at **www.ncbi.nlm.nih.gov/pubmed**. Type "aphasia" (or synonyms) into the search box, and click "Go." The following is the type of output you can expect from PubMed for "aphasia" (hyperlinks

- **An on-line analysis of syntactic processing in Broca's and Wernicke's aphasia.**
  Author(s): Zurif E, Swinney D, Prather P, Solomon J, Bushell C.
  Source: Brain and Language. 1993 October; 45(3): 448-64.
  http://www.ncbi.nlm.nih.gov:80/entrez/query.fcgi?cmd=Retrieve&db=PubMed&list_uids=8269334&dopt=Abstract

- **Developmental aphasia: impaired rate of non-verbal processing as a function of sensory modality.**
  Author(s): Tallal P, Piercy M.

---

[22] PubMed was developed by the National Center for Biotechnology Information (NCBI) at the National Library of Medicine (NLM) at the National Institutes of Health (NIH). The PubMed database was developed in conjunction with publishers of biomedical literature as a search tool for accessing literature citations and linking to full-text journal articles at Web sites of participating publishers. Publishers that participate in PubMed supply NLM with their citations electronically prior to or at the time of publication.

Source: Neuropsychologia. 1973 October; 11(4): 389-98. No Abstract Available.

http://www.ncbi.nlm.nih.gov:80/entrez/query.fcgi?cmd=Retrieve&db= PubMed&list_uids=4758181&dopt=Abstract

- **Family adjustment to aphasia.**
  Author(s): Davis GA.
  Source: Asha. 1990 November; 32(11): 63-4. No Abstract Available.
  http://www.ncbi.nlm.nih.gov:80/entrez/query.fcgi?cmd=Retrieve&db= PubMed&list_uids=2282087&dopt=Abstract

- **Singing as therapy for apraxia of speech and aphasia: report of a case.**
  Author(s): Keith RL, Aronson AE.
  Source: Brain and Language. 1975 October; 2(4): 483-8. No Abstract Available.
  http://www.ncbi.nlm.nih.gov:80/entrez/query.fcgi?cmd=Retrieve&db= PubMed&list_uids=1218380&dopt=Abstract

Vocabulary Builder

Accommodation: Adjustment, especially that of the eye for various distances. [EU]

Agnosia: Loss of the ability to comprehend the meaning or recognize the importance of various forms of stimulation that cannot be attributed to impairment of a primary sensory modality. Tactile agnosia is characterized by an inability to perceive the shape and nature of an object by touch alone, despite unimpaired sensation to light touch, position, and other primary sensory modalities. [NIH]

Amphetamine: A powerful central nervous system stimulant and sympathomimetic. Amphetamine has multiple mechanisms of action including blocking uptake of adrenergics and dopamine, stimulation of release of monamines, and inhibiting monoamine oxidase. Amphetamine is also a drug of abuse and a psychotomimetic. The l- and the d,l-forms are included here. The l-form has less central nervous system activity but stronger cardiovascular effects. The d-form is dextroamphetamine. [NIH]

Cerebral: Of or pertaining of the cerebrum or the brain. [EU]

Cortex: The outer layer of an organ or other body structure, as distinguished from the internal substance. [EU]

Curative: Tending to overcome disease and promote recovery. [EU]

Encephalopathy: Any degenerative disease of the brain. [EU]

Extremity: A limb; an arm or leg (membrum); sometimes applied specifically to a hand or foot. [EU]

Hemiplegia: Paralysis of one side of the body. [EU]

Hyperbaric: Characterized by greater than normal pressure or weight; applied to gases under greater than atmospheric pressure, as hyperbaric oxygen, or to a solution of greater specific gravity than another taken as a standard of reference. [EU]

Infarction: 1. the formation of an infarct. 2. an infarct. [EU]

Lesion: Any pathological or traumatic discontinuity of tissue or loss of function of a part. [EU]

Localization: 1. the determination of the site or place of any process or lesion. 2. restriction to a circumscribed or limited area. 3. prelocalization. [EU]

Mobility: Capability of movement, of being moved, or of flowing freely. [EU]

Neural: 1. pertaining to a nerve or to the nerves. 2. situated in the region of the spinal axis, as the neutral arch. [EU]

Norepinephrine: Precursor of epinephrine that is secreted by the adrenal medulla and is a widespread central and autonomic neurotransmitter. Norepinephrine is the principal transmitter of most postganglionic sympathetic fibers and of the diffuse projection system in the brain arising from the locus ceruleus. It is also found in plants and is used pharmacologically as a sympathomimetic. [NIH]

Parietal: 1. of or pertaining to the walls of a cavity. 2. pertaining to or located near the parietal bone, as the parietal lobe. [EU]

Pharmacologic: Pertaining to pharmacology or to the properties and reactions of drugs. [EU]

Posterior: Situated in back of, or in the back part of, or affecting the back or dorsal surface of the body. In lower animals, it refers to the caudal end of the body. [EU]

Prosthesis: An artificial substitute for a missing body part, such as an arm or leg, eye or tooth, used for functional or cosmetic reasons, or both. [EU]

Socialization: The training or molding of an individual through various relationships, educational agencies, and social controls, which enables him to become a member of a particular society. [NIH]

Symptomatology: 1. that branch of medicine with treats of symptoms; the systematic discussion of symptoms. 2. the combined symptoms of a disease. [EU]

CHAPTER 5. BOOKS ON APHASIA

Overview

This chapter provides bibliographic book references relating to aphasia. You have many options to locate books on aphasia. The simplest method is to go to your local bookseller and inquire about titles that they have in stock or can special order for you. Some patients, however, feel uncomfortable approaching their local booksellers and prefer online sources (e.g. **www.amazon.com** and **www.bn.com**). In addition to online booksellers, excellent sources for book titles on aphasia include the Combined Health Information Database and the National Library of Medicine. Once you have found a title that interests you, visit your local public or medical library to see if it is available for loan.

Book Summaries: Federal Agencies

The Combined Health Information Database collects various book abstracts from a variety of healthcare institutions and federal agencies. To access these summaries, go to **http://chid.nih.gov/detail/detail.html**. You will need to use the "Detailed Search" option. To find book summaries, use the drop boxes at the bottom of the search page where "You may refine your search by." Select the dates and language you prefer. For the format option, select "Monograph/Book." Now type "aphasia" (or synonyms) into the "For these words:" box. You will only receive results on books. You should check back periodically with this database which is updated every 3 months. The following is a typical result when searching for books on aphasia:

- **Assessment of Aphasia and Related Disorders. 2nd Ed**

  Source: Malvern, PA: Lea and Febiger. 1983. [134 p.].

Contact: Available from Lea and Febiger. 200 Chester Field Parkway, Malvern, PA 19355-9725. (610) 251-2230. PRICE: $47.00 for complete package including the Boston Diagnostic Aphasia Examination Booklet, 16 Test Stimulus Cards, Boston Naming Test, and Boston Naming Test Scoring Booklet. ISBN: 0812109015.

Summary: This book offers some insights into the assessment of aphasia and related disorders that can serve as a bridge to relating test scores to the common aphasic syndromes recognized by neurologists. This book's opening two chapters describes aphasic disorders and the goals and rationale of the assessment procedure. Chapter 3 cites the statistical data available up to 1982. Chapter 4 describes the test procedure, subtest by subtest, and is intended to serve as an instruction manual for the examiner. Chapter 5 describes additional, unstandardized, special language testing procedures, some of which are being investigated and others that are used informally at the Boston University Aphasia Research Center. Chapter 6 describes a supplementary nonverbal battery covering apraxia and the quantitative, visuospatial, and somatognostic problems that, in addition to language, are so often implicated. Chapter 7 describes the major aphasic syndromes, discusses some of the rare pure forms of selective aphasia, and shows how each pattern is reflected in the Aphasia Test score profile, with the help of selected case summaries. This book includes the Boston Diagnostic Aphasia Examination and 16 stimulus cards.

- **Coping with Aphasia**

Source: San Diego, CA: Singular Publishing Group, Inc. 1998. 462 p.

Contact: Available from Singular Publishing Group, Inc. 401 West 'A' Street, Suite 325, San Diego, CA 92101-7904. (800) 521-8545 or (619) 238-6777. Fax (800) 774-8398 or (619) 238-6789. E-mail: singpub@singpub.com. Website: www.singpub.com. PRICE: $18.95 plus shipping and handling. ISBN: 1879105756.

Summary: This book explains the nature of aphasia, a communication disorder that can disrupt the lives of not only those with aphasia but their families as well. The author describes in clear detail what the person with aphasia confronts over a duration of several years, and provides constructive advice to people with aphasia, their loved ones, caregivers, and therapists. Fourteen chapters cover a definition of aphasia; what to expect; the stages of hospitalization, rehabilitation, and formal care; how the brain handles speech, language, and communication changes due to aphasia; the causes of aphasia; what may accompany aphasia and what can be done to minimize further injury; and living life productively in spite of aphasia. The book includes four appendices: a glossary of terms;

a list of printed resource materials; a list of national, state, and international agencies associated with stroke and aphasia; and a list of agencies or businesses providing technical or treatment-related assistance, materials, or aids. The book concludes with a subject index.

- **Approaches to the Treatment of Aphasia**

  Source: San Diego, CA: Singular Publishing Group, Inc. 1998. 274 p.

  Contact: Available from Singular Publishing Group, Inc. 401 West 'A' Street, Suite 325, San Diego, CA 92101-7904. (800) 521-8545 or (619) 238-6777. Fax (800) 774-8398 or (619) 238-6789. E-mail: singpub@singpub.com. Website: www.singpub.com. PRICE: $49.95 plus shipping and handling. ISBN: 1565938410.

  Summary: This book is a collection of reports from clinicians about the clinical management of specific individuals with aphasia. The volume presents readers with an opportunity to eavesdrop on some highly experienced clinicians as they grapple with the very real problems of helping their particular patients. The eight cases were originally presented to other clinicians at a conference in Cody, Wyoming in October 1996. The introductory chapter reviews the historical perspective of using case studies, particularly in the field of aphasia therapy. The other eight chapters each offer one case study, covering issues including a case of aphasia, apraxia of speech, and apraxia of phonation; a strategy for improving oral naming in an individual with a phonological access impairment; a cognitive approach to treatment of an aphasic patient; an experimental treatment of sentence comprehension; treating sentence production in agrammatic aphasia; treatment for letter by letter reading; alexia without agraphia; and treating real life functionality in a couple coping with severe aphasia. A final chapter summarizes the impact on clinical care of a changing health care system. Most chapters conclude with a list of references and the book concludes with a subject index.

- **Adult Aphasia Rehabilitation**

  Source: Woburn, MA: Butterworth-Heinemann. 1996. 413 p.

  Contact: Available from Butterworth-Heinemann. 225 Wildwood Avenue, P.O. Box 4500, Woburn, MA 01801-2041. (617) 928-2500; Fax (617) 933-6333. PRICE: $47.50 plus shipping and handling. ISBN: 0750695358.

  Summary: This book focuses on topics of practical relevance to clinicians and advanced graduate students specializing in the rehabilitation of adults who have acquired aphasia. Twenty chapters cover medical and rehabilitation management, rehabilitation funding, clinical descriptions, language assessment, basic hearing assessment, the management of aphasic individuals from culturally and linguistically diverse populations, models for treatment, treatment of auditory comprehension impairment, rehabilitation of acquired reading disorders, treatment of naming and writing impairments, augmentative and alternative communication, psychological adjustment following stroke, planning rehabilitation services for rural and remote communities, and stroke prevention. The last chapter provides a resource guide for aphasia and stroke. A subject index concludes the volume.

- **Aphasia: A Clinical Perspective**

Source: New York, NY: Oxford University Press, Inc. 1996. 449 p.

Contact: Available from Oxford University Press, Inc. 200 Madison Avenue, New York, NY 10016. (800) 334-4249 or (212) 679-7300. PRICE: $49.95 plus shipping and handling. ISBN: 0195089340.

Summary: This book presents an integrated analysis of the language disturbances associated with brain pathology. In examining the different types of aphasia, the authors combine two clinical approaches: the neurological and the neuropsychological. Although they stress the clinical aspects of aphasia syndromes, they also review assessment techniques, linguistic analyses, problems of aphasia classification, and frequently occurring related disorders such as alexia, agraphia, acalculia, and anomia. In addition, they examine commonly encountered speech disorders, neurobehavioral and psychiatric problems commonly associated with aphasia, and the language characteristics of aging and dementia. Rehabilitation and recovery are discussed, and a neural basis for aphasia and related problems is proposed. Topics of specific interest to communication disorders include the lateralization of language function, the language area in the brain, childhood language disorders, developmental language disorders, aphasia in special languages (i.e., sign language), vascular disorders, brain trauma, neoplasms, infections, miscellaneous causes of aphasia, localization techniques, conduction aphasia, Wernicke aphasia, and clinical testing for aphasia. A subject index concludes the volume. 1237 references. (AA-M).

- **Aphasia Treatment: World Perspectives**

Source: San Diego, Ca: Singular Publishing Group, Inc. 1993. 377 p.

Contact: Available from Singular Publishing Group, Inc. 401 West 'A' Street, Suite 325, San Diego, CA 92101-7904. (800) 521-8545 or (619) 238-6777. Fax (800) 774-8398 or (619) 238-6789. E-mail: singpub@singpub.com.

Website: www.singpub.com. PRICE: $55.00 plus shipping and handling. ISBN: 1879105640.

Summary: This book is written by a group of international experts in aphasia treatment who describe their approaches to aphasia rehabilitation. Fourteen chapters cover therapy for aphasia in Italy, aphasia therapy in South Africa, aphasia therapy in Aachen, Germany, hypothesis testing and aphasia therapy (England), perspectives on aphasia intervention in French speaking Canada, the re-education of aphasics (Belgium), the concept of holistic rehabilitation of persons with aphasia (Poland), aphasia treatment in Japan, training conversation partners for aphasic adults, a multidisciplinary approach to aphasia therapy (the Netherlands), aphasia rehabilitation (Australia), different routes to aphasia therapy (Switzerland), psychosocial aspects in the treatment of adult aphasics and their families (Germany), and clinical intervention for aphasia in the United States. In describing treatment approaches in their respective countries, the authors find a common theme regarding pragmatic issues as well as a shared interest in cognitive neuropsychology. Many of the chapters refer to the World Health Organization's distinctions between disability, impairment, and handicap. Each chapter contains an extensive list of references. A subject index concludes the volume.

- **Living with Aphasia: Psychosocial Issues**

Source: San Diego, CA: Singular Publishing Group, Inc. 1992. 305 p.

Contact: Available from Singular Publishing Group, Inc. 401 West 'A' Street, Suite 325, San Diego, CA 92101-7904. (800) 521-8545 or (619) 238-6777. Fax (800) 774-8398 or (619) 238-6789. E-mail: singpub@singpub.com. Website: www.singpub.com. PRICE: $47.50 plus shipping and handling. ISBN: 1565930673.

Summary: This book explores the psychosocial issues of living with aphasia. Sixteen chapters are presented in five sections: introspection; the person with aphasia; the person with aphasia and treatment; the family; and the person with aphasia and society. Specific topics covered include self-awareness of the problem of aphasia; the physical experience of the person with aphasia; the psychological effects of aphasia; aphasia and artistic creation; the dynamics of speech therapy; typical behavior of persons with aphasia and their families; the bilingual person with aphasia; workplace considerations; legal issues; ethical-moral dilemmas in aphasia rehabilitation; and associations for persons with aphasia. The book includes extensive quotations from people with aphasia, as well as numerous case examples.

- **Acquired Aphasia. 2nd Ed**

  Source: Orlando, FL: Academic Press, Inc. 1991. 614 p.

  Contact: Available from Academic Press, Inc. 6277 Sea Harbor Drive, Orlando, FL 32887. (800) 245-8744; Fax (800) 874-6418. PRICE: $64.95 plus shipping and handling. ISBN: 0126193215.

  Summary: This textbook brings together the writing of some well known workers in the field of aphasia. Sixteen chapters cover historical perspectives, signs of aphasia, neuroanatomical correlates of the aphasias, assessment, phonological aspects of aphasia, lexical deficits, sentence processing, explanations for the concept of apraxia of speech, aphasia-related disorders, intelligence and aphasia, artistry and aphasia, language in aging and dementia, acquired aphasia in children, aphasia after head injury, the psychological and social sequelae of aphasia, and recovery and rehabilitation considerations. Each chapter includes extensive references, and the text concludes with a subject index. The editor notes that the scope of this volume does not permit a review of the techniques and practice of aphasia therapy, but instead outlines broad principles.

- **Understanding Stroke and Aphasia**

  Source: Austin, TX: Pro-Ed, Inc. 1990. 96 p.

  Contact: Available from Pro-Ed, Inc. 8700 Shoal Creek Boulevard, Austin, TX 78757-6897. (512) 451-3246; Fax (800) FXPROED or (512) 451-8542; http://www.proedinc.com. PRICE: $14.00 plus shipping and handling. Order Number 1490.

  Summary: This book provides information for patients and families who are adapting to changes caused by stroke and aphasia. The author, using a question and answer format, discusses definitions, causes, prognosis, nonlanguage problems associated with aphasia, and residual problems following a stroke and aphasia. The author also provides specific suggestions for activities of daily living and for coping with the psychosocial factors. A glossary and resource list are included. 35 references.

- **Pathways: Moving Beyond Stroke and Aphasia**

  Source: Detroit, MI: Wayne State University Press. 1990. 198 p.

  Contact: Available from Wayne State University Press. Leonard N. Simons Building, 4809 Woodward Avenue, Detroit, MI 48201-1309. (800) 978-7323 or (313) 577-6120; Fax (313) 577-6131. PRICE: $34.95 plus shipping and handling. ISBN 0814320740.

Summary: This book portrays the experiences of six Detroit-area families when stroke and aphasia intrude on their lives. The book explores issues, such as physical and emotional reactions to stroke and aphasia and the responses of other family members to stroke and aphasia, that are universal to those coping with these crises. There is also information about prescription drugs, medical tests, and suggestions for other resources. Includes bibliographic references.

- **Speech-Language Treatment of the Aphasias Workbook II: Treatment Materials for Oral Expression and Written Expression**

Source: Frederick, MD: Aspen Publishers, Inc. 1989. 283 p.

Contact: Available from Aspen Publishers, Inc. 7201 McKinney Circle, P.O. Box 990, Frederick, MD 21701-9782. (800) 638-8437 or (301) 417-7500; Fax (301) 417-7650. PRICE: $51.00 plus shipping and handling. ISBN: 0834200805.

Summary: Directed toward clinicians, this book of aphasia treatment materials was developed to accompany the source book 'Speech/Language Treatment of the Aphasias: An Integrated Clinical Approach.' This workbook is intended to be used for planning and conducting a comprehensive treatment program. It includes student/clinician exercises to build oral and written expression skills in patients with aphasia. Twelve units provide sentence completion tasks, responsive naming tasks, conversational tasks (role playing tasks for group treatment), anagrams, visual closure, single-word categorization, sentence completion tasks, written retrieval sentence completion tasks, definitions, correcting misspelled words in sentences, correcting misspelled words in paragraphs, and higher-level syntactical structures.

- **Speech-Language Treatment of the Aphasias Workbook I: Treatment Materials for Auditory Comprehension and Reading Comprehension**

Source: Frederick, MD: Aspen Publishers, Inc. 1989. 377 p.

Contact: Available from Aspen Publishers, Inc. 7201 McKinney Circle, P.O. Box 990, Frederick, MD 21701-9782. (800) 638-8437 or (301) 417-7500; Fax (301) 417-7650. PRICE: $51.00 plus shipping and handling. ISBN: 0834200791.

Summary: Directed toward clinicians, this book of aphasia treatment materials was developed to accompany the source book 'Speech/Language Treatment of the Aphasias: An Integrated Clinical Approach.' This workbook is intended to be used for planning and conducting a comprehensive treatment program. It includes student/clinician exercises to build auditory and reading comprehension skills in patients with aphasia. Twenty-four units provide activities for working on complex directions and factual questions, interpreting metaphorical language, complex connected speech, discriminating between real and nonsense words, correct versus incorrect vocabulary, word order, verb form, word choice, question form, negatives, and grammatical forms, identifying a designated WH constituent, WH questions, categorizing low-frequency words, identifying semantic constituents, simple paragraph comprehension, comprehending unfamiliar short paragraphs, functional paragraph material, reordering sentences, and comprehending complex paragraphs.

Book Summaries: Online Booksellers

Commercial Internet-based booksellers, such as Amazon.com and Barnes & Noble.com, offer summaries which have been supplied by each title's publisher. Some summaries also include customer reviews. Your local bookseller may have access to in-house and commercial databases that index all published books (e.g. Books in Print®). The following have been recently listed with online booksellers as relating to aphasia (sorted alphabetically by title; follow the hyperlink to view more details at Amazon.com):

- **Administrative Manual for the Minnesota Test for Differential Diagnosis of Aphasia** by Hildred Schuell (1965); ISBN: 0816611998; http://www.amazon.com/exec/obidos/ASIN/0816611998/icongroupin terna

- **Adult Aphasia** by Jon Eisenson (1983); ISBN: 0130087718; http://www.amazon.com/exec/obidos/ASIN/0130087718/icongroupin terna

- **Adult Aphasia.** by Harvey. Halpern (1972); ISBN: 0672612801; http://www.amazon.com/exec/obidos/ASIN/0672612801/icongroupin terna

- **Adult Has Aphasia** (1983); ISBN: 081340827X; http://www.amazon.com/exec/obidos/ASIN/081340827X/icongroupi nterna

- **Adult Has Aphasia** by Daniel R. Boone (1983); ISBN: 0813423422; http://www.amazon.com/exec/obidos/ASIN/0813423422/icongroupin terna

- **Aphasia** by Libby Kumin (1978); ISBN: 0822018160; http://www.amazon.com/exec/obidos/ASIN/0822018160/icongroupin terna

- **Aphasia** by Frederic L Darley (1982); ISBN: 0721628796; http://www.amazon.com/exec/obidos/ASIN/0721628796/icongroupin terna

- **Aphasia and Associated Disorders : Taxonomy, Localization and Recovery** by Andrew Kertesz (1979); ISBN: 0808911937; http://www.amazon.com/exec/obidos/ASIN/0808911937/icongroupin terna

- **Aphasia Handbook for Adults and Children** by Aleen Agranowitz (1975); ISBN: 9992057742; http://www.amazon.com/exec/obidos/ASIN/9992057742/icongroupin terna

- **Aphasia Rehabilitation : An Auditory and Verbal Task Hierarchy** by Deborah Ross, Sara Spencer (1980); ISBN: 0398040311; http://www.amazon.com/exec/obidos/ASIN/0398040311/icongroupin terna

- **Aphasia Theory and Therapy: Selected Lectures and Papers of Hildred Schuell** by Hildred. Schuell (1983); ISBN: 081912768X; http://www.amazon.com/exec/obidos/ASIN/081912768X/icongroupi nterna

- **Aphasia Therapy Manual** by Joseph C. Aurelia (1974); ISBN: 0813421128; http://www.amazon.com/exec/obidos/ASIN/0813421128/icongroupin terna

- **Aphasia, Alexia and Agraphia** by David Frank Benson (1980); ISBN: 0443080410; http://www.amazon.com/exec/obidos/ASIN/0443080410/icongroupin terna

- **Aphasia, My World Alone** (1979); ISBN: 0814316468; http://www.amazon.com/exec/obidos/ASIN/0814316468/icongroupin terna

- **Card Materials for the Minnesota Test for Differential Diagnosis of Aphasia/Set 2 Packs** by Hildred Schuell, Lawrence Benson (1965); ISBN: 0816612005; http://www.amazon.com/exec/obidos/ASIN/0816612005/icongroupin terna

- **Communication Disorders** by Rieber (1981); ISBN: 030640527X; http://www.amazon.com/exec/obidos/ASIN/030640527X/icongroupi nterna

- **Cry Babel: The Nightmare of Aphasia and a Courageous Woman's Struggle to Rebuild Her Life** by April Oursler Armstrong (1979); ISBN:

0385135297;
http://www.amazon.com/exec/obidos/ASIN/0385135297/icongroupin
terna

- **Differential Diagnosis of Aphasia With the Minnesota Test** by Hildred Schuell, Joyce W. Sefer (1973); ISBN: 0816606730;
http://www.amazon.com/exec/obidos/ASIN/0816606730/icongroupin
terna

- **Graduated Language Training Treatment Manual for Patients With Aphasia and Children With Language Deficiencies** by Robert L. Keith (1980); ISBN: 0933014570;
http://www.amazon.com/exec/obidos/ASIN/0933014570/icongroupin
terna

- **Guide to Understanding Aphasia** by William O. and Greenberg, Bonita R. Haynes (1976); ISBN: 0813418054;
http://www.amazon.com/exec/obidos/ASIN/0813418054/icongroupin
terna

- **Language Acquisition and Language Breakdown : Parallels and Divergencies** by Baltimore (1978); ISBN: 0801819482;
http://www.amazon.com/exec/obidos/ASIN/0801819482/icongroupin
terna

- **Language Development and Aphasia in Children: New Essays and a Translation of Kindersprasce and Asphasie** by W. Rieber (1980); ISBN: 0125882807;
http://www.amazon.com/exec/obidos/ASIN/0125882807/icongroupin
terna

- **Language Handicaps in Adults** by William H. Perkins (Editor) (1983); ISBN: 0865770905;
http://www.amazon.com/exec/obidos/ASIN/0865770905/icongroupin
terna

- **Linguistic Investigation of Aphasia** by Ruth Lesser (1978); ISBN: 0713159669;
http://www.amazon.com/exec/obidos/ASIN/0713159669/icongroupin
terna

- **Management of Aphasia** by Yvan Lebrun, Richard Hoops (1978); ISBN: 902650280X;
http://www.amazon.com/exec/obidos/ASIN/902650280X/icongroupi
nterna

- **Neologistic Jargon Aphasia (Neurolinguistics Series: Vol 3)** by H. W. Buckingham (1976); ISBN: 9026502273;

http://www.amazon.com/exec/obidos/ASIN/9026502273/icongroupin
terna

- **Perspectives In Neurolinguistics : The Bilingual Brain : Neuropsychological and Neurolinguistic Aspects of Bilingualism** by Martin L. Albert, Loraine K. Obler (1978); ISBN: 0120487500; http://www.amazon.com/exec/obidos/ASIN/0120487500/icongroupin terna

- **Problems of Aphasia** by Yvan Lebrun, Richard Hoops (1979); ISBN: 9026503091; http://www.amazon.com/exec/obidos/ASIN/9026503091/icongroupin terna

- **Readings on Aphasia in Bilinguals and Polyglots** by Michel Paradis (Editor) (1983); ISBN: 2891440684; http://www.amazon.com/exec/obidos/ASIN/2891440684/icongroupin terna

- **Recovery with Aphasia: The Aftermath of My Stroke** by Claude Scott Moss (1972); ISBN: 0252002717; http://www.amazon.com/exec/obidos/ASIN/0252002717/icongroupin terna

- **Silent Victory** by Carmen McBride (1969); ISBN: 0911012036; http://www.amazon.com/exec/obidos/ASIN/0911012036/icongroupin terna

- **Sourcebook for Aphasia : A Guide to Family Activities and Community Resources** by Susan Howell Brubaker (1981); ISBN: 0814316972; http://www.amazon.com/exec/obidos/ASIN/0814316972/icongroupin terna

- **Speech After Stroke : A Manual for the Speech Pathologist and the Family Member** by Stephanie Stryker (1980); ISBN: 0398041229; http://www.amazon.com/exec/obidos/ASIN/0398041229/icongroupin terna

- **Stroke : A Doctor's Personal Story of His Recovery** by Charles Clay Dahlberg (1977); ISBN: 0393087204; http://www.amazon.com/exec/obidos/ASIN/0393087204/icongroupin terna

- **Studies on Child Language and Aphasia (Janua Linguarum, Minor, No 114)** by Roman Jakobson (1971); ISBN: 9027916403; http://www.amazon.com/exec/obidos/ASIN/9027916403/icongroupin terna

- **The Western Aphasia Battery : Test Booklet** by Andrew Kertesz (1982);
  ISBN: 0808914553;
  http://www.amazon.com/exec/obidos/ASIN/0808914553/icongroupin
  terna

- **The Western Aphasia Battery : Test Cards** by Andrew Kertesz (1982);
  ISBN: 0808914561;
  http://www.amazon.com/exec/obidos/ASIN/0808914561/icongroupin
  terna

- **The Western Aphasia Battery : Test Manual** by Andrew Kertesz (1982);
  ISBN: 0808914545;
  http://www.amazon.com/exec/obidos/ASIN/0808914545/icongroupin
  terna

- **Traumatic Aphasia : Its Syndromes, Psychology and Treatment (Janua Linguarum Series Major No 5)** by A.R. Luria (1970); ISBN: 902790717X;
  http://www.amazon.com/exec/obidos/ASIN/902790717X/icongroupi
  nterna

- **Treatise on Aphasia and Other Speech Defects** by Henry C. Bastian
  (1978); ISBN: 0404608515;
  http://www.amazon.com/exec/obidos/ASIN/0404608515/icongroupin
  terna

The National Library of Medicine Book Index

The National Library of Medicine at the National Institutes of Health has a massive database of books published on healthcare and biomedicine. Go to the following Internet site, **http://locatorplus.gov/,** and then select "Search LOCATORplus." Once you are in the search area, simply type "aphasia" (or synonyms) into the search box, and select "books only." From there, results can be sorted by publication date, author, or relevance. The following was recently catalogued by the National Library of Medicine:[23]

---

[23] In addition to LOCATORPlus, in collaboration with authors and publishers, the National Center for Biotechnology Information (NCBI) is adapting biomedical books for the Web. The books may be accessed in two ways: (1) by searching directly using any search term or phrase (in the same way as the bibliographic database PubMed), or (2) by following the links to PubMed abstracts. Each PubMed abstract has a "Books" button that displays a facsimile of the abstract in which some phrases are hypertext links. These phrases are also found in the books available at NCBI. Click on hyperlinked results in the list of books in which the phrase is found. Currently, the majority of the links are between the books and PubMed. In the future, more links will be created between the books and other types of information, such as gene and protein sequences and macromolecular structures. See **http://www.ncbi.nlm.nih.gov/entrez/query.fcgi?db=Books.**

- **Acquired neurogenic communication disorders: a clinical perspective.** Author: edited by Ilias Papathanasiou; Year: 2000; London; Philadelphia: Whurr Publishers, 2000; ISBN: 1861561113
  http://www.amazon.com/exec/obidos/ASIN/1861561113/icongroupin terna

- **Aphasia: a social approach.** Author: Lesley Jordan and Wendy Kaiser; Year: 1996; London; New York: Chapman & Hall, 1996; ISBN: 041249700X (alk. paper)
  http://www.amazon.com/exec/obidos/ASIN/041249700X/icongroupi nterna

- **Aphasia and language: theory to practice.** Author: edited by Stephen E. Nadeau, Leslie J. Gonzalez Rothi, Bruce Crosson; Year: 2000; New York: Guilford Press, c2000; ISBN: 1572305819 (alk. paper)
  http://www.amazon.com/exec/obidos/ASIN/1572305819/icongroupin terna

- **Aphasia as a challenge to AAC.** Author: ed., Marketta Kortesmaa; Year: 1996; Turku, Finland: Stroke and <STRONG><I>Aphasia</I></STRONG> Federation, 1996; ISBN: 9525058034

- **Aphasia in atypical populations.** Author: edited by Patrick Coppens, Yvan Lebrun, Anna Basso; Year: 1998; Mahwah, N.J.: Lawrence Erlbaum Associates, 1998; ISBN: 0805817387 (alk. paper)
  http://www.amazon.com/exec/obidos/ASIN/0805817387/icongroupin terna

- **Aphasiology: disorders and clinical practice.** Author: G. Albyn Davis; Year: 2000; Boston: Allyn and Bacon, c2000; ISBN: 0205298346 (hardcover)
  http://www.amazon.com/exec/obidos/ASIN/0205298346/icongroupin terna

- **Approaches to the treatment of aphasia.** Author: edited by Nancy Helm-Estabrooks and Audrey L. Holland; Year: 1998; San Diego: Singular Pub. Group, c1998; ISBN: 1565938410
  http://www.amazon.com/exec/obidos/ASIN/1565938410/icongroupin terna

- **Assessment of aphasia and related disorders.** Author: Harold Goodglass; with the collaboration of Edith Kaplan and Barbara Barresi; Year: 2001; Philadelphia: Lippincott Williams & Wilkins, c2001; ISBN: 068330559X
  http://www.amazon.com/exec/obidos/ASIN/068330559X/icongroupi nterna

- **Beyond aphasia: therapies for living with communication disability.**
Author: Carole Pound... [et al.]; Year: 2000; Bicester, Oxon, UK: Winslow Press, 2000; ISBN: 0863882307
http://www.amazon.com/exec/obidos/ASIN/0863882307/icongroupin terna

- **Brain and language: seminar proceedings.** Author: editors, P.A. Suresh, Annie Monsy, S. Maya; Year: 1994; Thiruvananthapuram: International School of Dravidian Linguistics, [1994]; ISBN: 8185692122
http://www.amazon.com/exec/obidos/ASIN/8185692122/icongroupin terna

- **Children with language disorders.** Author: Janet Lees, Shelagh Urwin; Year: 1997; London: Whurr Publishers, 1997; ISBN: 1861560265

- **Coping with aphasia.** Author: Jon G. Lyon; Year: 1998; San Diego: Singular Pub. Group, c1998; ISBN: 1879105756
http://www.amazon.com/exec/obidos/ASIN/1879105756/icongroupin terna

- **Exploring the history of neuropsychology: selected papers.** Author: Arthur Benton; with an introduction by Kenneth M. Adams; Year: 2000; Oxford; New York: Oxford University Press, 2000; ISBN: 0195138082 (alk. paper)
http://www.amazon.com/exec/obidos/ASIN/0195138082/icongroupin terna

- **Freud and his aphasia book: language and the sources of psychoanalysis.** Author: Valerie D. Greenberg; Year: 1997; Ithaca, N.Y.: Cornell University Press, 1997; ISBN: 0801432847 (hardcover: alk. paper)
http://www.amazon.com/exec/obidos/ASIN/0801432847/icongroupin terna

- **Grammatical disorders in aphasia: a neurolinguistic perspective.** Author: edited by Roelien Bastiaanse and Yosef Grodzinsky; Year: 2000; London; Philadelphia: Whurr Publishers, 2000; ISBN: 1861561350
http://www.amazon.com/exec/obidos/ASIN/1861561350/icongroupin terna

- **Introduction to group treatment for aphasia: design and management.** Author: Robert C. Marshall; Year: 1999; Boston: Butterworth-Heinemann, c1999; ISBN: 0750670134 (alk. paper)
http://www.amazon.com/exec/obidos/ASIN/0750670134/icongroupin terna

- **Introduction to neurogenic communication disorders.** Author: Robert H. Brookshire; Year: 1997; St. Louis: Mosby, c1997; ISBN: 0815110146
http://www.amazon.com/exec/obidos/ASIN/0815110146/icongroupin terna

- **Language intervention strategies in aphasia and related neurogenic communication disorders.** Author: editor, Roberta Chapey; Year: 2001; Philadelphia: Lippincott Williams & Wilkins, c2001; ISBN: 0781721334
  http://www.amazon.com/exec/obidos/ASIN/0781721334/icongroupinterna

- **Manual of cooperative group treatment for aphasia.** Author: [edited by] Jan R. Avent; Year: 1997; Boston: Butterworth-Heinemann, c1997; ISBN: 0750699213 (alk. paper)
  http://www.amazon.com/exec/obidos/ASIN/0750699213/icongroupinterna

- **Neurobehavior of language and cognition: studies of normal aging and brain damage: honoring Martin L. Albert.** Author: edited by Lisa Tabor Connor, Loraine K. Obler; Year: 2000; Boston: Kluwer Academic Publishers, c2000; ISBN: 0792378776 (alk. paper)
  http://www.amazon.com/exec/obidos/ASIN/0792378776/icongroupinterna

- **Proceedings of the Fifth National Aphasiology Symposium of Australia, Newcastle, October 3-4, 1997.** Author: proceedings edited by Alison Ferguson; Year: 1998; Callaghan Newcastle, NSW: University of Newcastle, c1998; ISBN: 0752910402

- **Spoken word production and its breakdown in aphasia.** Author: Lyndsey Nickels; Year: 1997; Hove, East Sussex, UK: Psychology Press, c1997; ISBN: 0863774660
  http://www.amazon.com/exec/obidos/ASIN/0863774660/icongroupinterna

- **Talking about aphasia: living with loss of language after stroke.** Author: Susie Parr, Sally Byng, and Sue Gilpin; with Chris Ireland; Year: 1997; Buckingham; Philadelphia: Open University Press, 1997; ISBN: 0335199372 (hb)
  http://www.amazon.com/exec/obidos/ASIN/0335199372/icongroupinterna

- **Transcortical aphasias.** Author: Marcelo L. Berthier; Year: 1999; Hove, East Sussex, UK: Psychology Press, c1999; ISBN: 0863778402 (Hbk)
  http://www.amazon.com/exec/obidos/ASIN/0863778402/icongroupinterna

- **Treatise on aphasia and other speech defects.** Author: by H. Charlton Bastian ...; with illustrations; Year: 1898; New York: D. Appleton and Company, 1898

Chapters on Aphasia

Frequently, aphasia will be discussed within a book, perhaps within a specific chapter. In order to find chapters that are specifically dealing with aphasia, an excellent source of abstracts is the Combined Health Information Database. You will need to limit your search to book chapters and aphasia using the "Detailed Search" option. Go directly to the following hyperlink: **http://chid.nih.gov/detail/detail.html**. To find book chapters, use the drop boxes at the bottom of the search page where "You may refine your search by." Select the dates and language you prefer, and the format option "Book Chapter." By making these selections and typing in "aphasia" (or synonyms) into the "For these words:" box, you will only receive results on chapters in books. The following is a typical result when searching for book chapters on aphasia:

- **Differentiating Dementia and Aphasia**

    Source: in Bayles, K.A.; Kaszniak, A.W. Communication and Cognition in Normal Aging and Dementia. Boston, MA: College-Hill Press. 1987. p. 179-204.

    Contact: This publication may be available from your local medical library. Call for information. ISBN: 0316083976.

    Summary: This chapter summarizes and discusses available evidence for differentiating between aphasia, defined as a loss of expression or understanding caused by brain damage, and dementia. Aphasia is considered a general condition with many subtypes, one of which is the aphasia of dementia. Many experts apply the term aphasia to the language problems of dementia patients. Major attention is given to the nature and results of test used in the differential diagnosis of dementia and aphasia. Consideration also is given to: differentiating criteria; opposition to calling the communication impairment of dementia patients, aphasia; and considerations of what communication problems of the dementia patient should be called. Data are included on the performance of dementia patients on different aphasia tests. It is concluded that, of those patients with classic aphasia syndromes, those with fluent aphasias and preserved repetition are more likely to be confused with Alzheimer's disease patients. Clinical implications with this topic are discussed. 78 references.

- **Aphasia**

    Source: in Vinson, B.P. Essentials for Speech-Language Pathologists. San Diego, CA: Singular Publishing Group. 2001. p. 81-98.

Contact: Available from Thomson Learning Group. P.O. Box 6904, Florence, KY 41022. (800) 842-3636. Fax (606) 647-5963. Website: www.singpub.com. Price: $49.95 plus shipping and handling. ISBN: 0769300715.

Summary: Aphasia is an impairment of the ability to comprehend and formulate language due to damage to the central nervous system . Aphasia does not include language deficits caused by dementia, motor dysfunction, or a sensory loss. This chapter on aphasia is from a textbook that is designed to help new professionals with the transition to clinical practice in speech language pathology. The author reviews the defining characteristics of aphasia and explains why speech language pathologists are involved in the assessment and treatment of persons with aphasia. Topics include the etiology of stroke; the timing of strokes; questions to guide the evaluation of patients with neurological deficits; the components of the assessment, including the neurological exam, and language testing, including naming, fluency, paraphasias, auditory comprehension, repetition skills, and standardized assessment tools. The author then discusses specific aphasia syndromes, including subcortical aphasias, fluent cortical aphasias, Wernicke's aphasia, conduction aphasia, and transcortical sensory aphasia; and nonfluent aphasias, including Broca's aphasia, transcortical motor aphasia, and global aphasia. The chapter then concludes with a discussion of treatment options. It discusses underlying processes; ways of promoting auditory comprehension; naming and functional communication; and specific treatment programs, including gestural reorganization, Melodic Intonation Therapy (MIT), Promoting Aphasics' Communication Effectiveness (PACE), the auditory stimulation approach, and Visual Action Therapy (VAT). 13 tables.

- **Proactive Management of Primary Progressive Aphasia**

Source: in Beukelman, D.R.; Yorkston, K.M.; Reichle, J., eds. Augmentative and Alternative Communication for Adults with Acquired Neurologic Disorders. Baltimore, MD: Paul H. Brookes Publishing Co. 2000. p. 305-337.

Contact: Available from Paul H. Brookes Publishing Co. P.O. Box 10624, Baltimore, MD 21285. (800) 638-3775. Fax (410) 337-8539. Website: www.brookespublishing.com. Price: $42.00 plus shipping and handling. ISBN: 1557664730.

Summary: The loss of speech in adulthood due to acquired neurologic disorders causes a person enormous life changes. This chapter on the use of augmentative and alternative communication (AAC) strategies for individuals with primary progressive aphasia (PPA) is from a textbook that explores the challenges these adults face during their transition, whether gradual or immediate, from speaking to using AAC. PPA is characterized by the gradual deterioration of language abilities in the context of preserved memory, judgement, insight, and visuospatial skills (which differentiates it from dementia or Alzheimer disease). The authors offer an approach to assist people with PPA and their families to make proactive adjustments concerning how they communicate and, in some respects, structure their lives. The intervention approach described is guided by the premise that as speech and language functioning decline, the communicative competency of the person with PPA can be maintained. The speech language pathologist is the principal health care professional responsible for assisting people with PPA, in part because there is presently no medical intervention available that can cure or decelerate the disease's progression. The chapter concludes with two vignettes demonstrating successful adaptation using AAC strategies. The authors reiterate the concept that negative life experiences can be successfully managed by reducing limitations in the physical and social environment and by participation in and enjoyment of valued activities. 1 figure. 4 tables. 58 references.

- **AAC and Aphasia: Cognitive-Linguistic Considerations**

Source: in Beukelman, D.R.; Yorkston, K.M.; Reichle, J., eds. Augmentative and Alternative Communication for Adults with Acquired Neurologic Disorders. Baltimore, MD: Paul H. Brookes Publishing Co. 2000. p. 339-374.

Contact: Available from Paul H. Brookes Publishing Co. P.O. Box 10624, Baltimore, MD 21285. (800) 638-3775. Fax (410) 337-8539. Website: www.brookespublishing.com. Price: $42.00 plus shipping and handling. ISBN: 1557664730.

Summary: The loss of speech in adulthood due to acquired neurologic disorders causes a person to confront enormous life changes. This chapter on the use of augmentative and alternative communication (AAC) strategies for individuals with aphasia is from a textbook that explores the challenges these adults face during their transition, whether gradual or immediate, from speaking to using AAC. Aphasia is a communication disorder that is typically acquired in a sudden manner by linguistically sophisticated adults. The neurologic injuries that cause aphasia are usually the result of a vascular accident (i.e., stroke) or injury to the left hemisphere of the brain. Aphasia is defined as complete or partial impairment of language comprehension. People with aphasia cannot consistently send or receive adequate linguistic signals. This inability can diminish their ability communicate effectively. For people with aphasia,

AAC design and implementation issues are different than those for people with motor impairments or cognitive developmental disabilities. The authors discuss historic intervention approaches for aphasia, how AAC strategies can be used in this population, basic premises about AAC learning and aphasia, the cognitive processes underlying aphasia, the cognitive linguistic demands of everyday communication situations, and methods of embedding cognitive linguistic support into AAC strategy training. The authors reiterate the importance of matching AAC strategies and equipment with the individual's needs and skills. 2 figures. 1 table. 68 references.

- **Intervention Planning for Adult Aphasia**

  Source: in Klein, H.B. and Moses, N. Intervention Planning for Adults with Communication Problems: A Guide for Clinical Practicum and Professional Practice. Needham Heights, MA: Allyn and Bacon. 1999. p. 197-270.

  Contact: Available from Allyn and Bacon. 160 Gould Street, Needham Heights, MA 02194. (800) 278-3525. Website: www.abacon.com. Price: $53.95. ISBN: 0205173853.

  Summary: Aphasia is an acquired organic communicative disorder that affects comprehension and production of spoken and written communication. This chapter on intervention planning for adult aphasia is from a textbook supporting students completing coursework for certification by the American Speech Language Hearing Association (ASHA), specifically the practicum hours in assessment and intervention with adult clients. Topics include the various categories of aphasia and associated communication characteristics; models of aphasia rehabilitation and how they are each applied to intervention planning; factors maintaining communication problems in adults with aphasia; and the formulation of a management plan that incorporates baseline data about language functioning and maintaining factors, and models of aphasia rehabilitation). The chapter offers a case study report of the course of intervention planning for an adult with aphasia. The chapter concludes with an appendix outlining a suggested hierarchy of difficulty for syntactic constructions by persons with aphasia. 15 tables. 132 references.

- **How Speech, Language, and Communication Change with Aphasia**

  Source: in Lyon, J.G. Coping with Aphasia. San Diego, CA: Singular Publishing Group, Inc. 1998. p. 313-328.

Contact: Available from Singular Publishing Group, Inc. 401 West 'A' Street, Suite 325, San Diego, CA 92101-7904. (800) 521-8545 or (619) 238-6777. Fax (800) 774-8398 or (619) 238-6789. E-mail: singpub@singpub.com. Website: www.singpub.com. Price: $18.95 plus shipping and handling. ISBN: 1879105756.

Summary: This chapter is from a book that explains the nature of aphasia, a communication disorder that can disrupt the lives of not only those with aphasia but their families as well. The author describes in clear detail what the person with aphasia confronts over a duration of several years, and provides constructive advice to people with aphasia, their loved ones, caregivers, and therapists. This chapter focuses on how speech, language, and communication change with aphasia. Topics include diagnostic tests that pinpoint these changes (identifying the site of the impairments), dealing with injury deep inside the brain, dealing with injury to the outer surface of the brain, identifying the type of aphasia, distinguishing between fluent and nonfluent aphasias, types of fluent aphasias (anomic, conduction, transcortical sensory, Wernicke's), types of nonfluent aphasias (transcortical, Broca's, global), picturing the actual injury to the brain, and speech impairments that are not aphasia (apraxia of speech and dysarthria). The author provides examples and encouragement. 3 figures. (AA-M).

- **Phonological Analysis of Apraxia of Speech in Broca's Aphasia**

Source: in Cannito, M.P.; Yorkston, K.M.; Beukelman, D.R., eds. Neuromotor Speech Disorders: Nature, Assessment, and Management. Baltimore, MD: Paul H. Brookes Publishing Company. 1998. p. 309-321.

Contact: Available from Paul H. Brookes Publishing Company. P.O. Box 10624, Baltimore, MD 21285-0624. (800) 638-3775. Fax (410) 337-8539. E-mail: custserv@pbrookes.com. Website: www.brookespublishing.com. Price: $44.95 plus shipping and handling. ISBN: 1557663262.

Summary: This chapter is from a textbook offering a compilation of research of interest to speech language pathologists, health care professionals, basic researchers, and students who treat or study pathologies of motor systems affecting speech communication. This chapter discusses the phonological analysis of apraxia of speech in Broca's aphasia. The authors present a study in which they describe the speech of 10 subjects with Broca's aphasia and apraxia of speech. The authors assume a phonological analytic vantage point to address the issue of potential linguistic explanations for observed speech output characteristics of apraxia in Broca's aphasia. Subjects had clinical characteristics of effortful, groping articulation; speech dysprosody; variable articulation errors; and other symptomatology congruent with the diagnosis of apraxia of speech. The results failed to reveal evidence that subjects with Broca's aphasia exhibit impairment in phonological ability. Error rates were low with limited use of phonological processes. The results support a motor programming interpretation of apraxia of speech as manifested in Broca's aphasia, as opposed to an underlying deficit at the phonological level of language processing. 4 figures. 2 tables. 23 references.

- **Power of One: Every Aphasia Treatment Case Is a Case Study**

Source: in Helm-Estabrooks, N. and Holland, A.L., eds. Approaches to the Treatment of Aphasia. San Diego, CA: Singular Publishing Group, Inc. 1998. p. 1-9.

Contact: Available from Singular Publishing Group, Inc. 401 West 'A' Street, Suite 325, San Diego, CA 92101-7904. (800) 521-8545 or (619) 238-6777. Fax (800) 774-8398 or (619) 238-6789. E-mail: singpub@singpub.com. Website: www.singpub.com. Price: $49.95 plus shipping and handling. ISBN: 1565938410.

Summary: This chapter is from a collection of reports from clinicians about the clinical management of specific individuals with aphasia. The volume presents readers with an opportunity to eavesdrop on some highly experienced clinicians as they grapple with the very real problems of helping their particular patients. This introductory chapter reviews the historical perspective of using case studies, particularly in the field of aphasia therapy. The author also discusses recent use of case studies, noting that since the early 1970s, there has been an explosion of literature pertaining to the treatment of aphasia. The author then introduces each of the eight case studies presented later in the book. The author concludes that case reports have played a strong role in the professional history of speech language pathologists and shall continue to do so in the future. 12 references.

- **Adults with Severe Aphasia**

Source: in Beukelman, D.R. and Mirenda, P. Augmentative and Alternative Communication: Management of Severe Communication Disorders in Children and Adults. 2nd ed. Baltimore, MD: Paul H. Brookes Publishing Co. 1998. p. 465-499.

Contact: Available from Paul H. Brookes Publishing Co. P.O. Box 10624, Baltimore, MD 21285. (800) 638-3775. Fax (410) 337-8539. Website: www.brookespublishing.com. Price: $59.95 plus shipping and handling. ISBN: 1557663335.

Summary: Aphasia is the impairment of an individual's ability to interpret and formulate language as a result of brain injury (most often, a stroke). This chapter on adults with severe aphasia is from a textbook that promotes a comprehensive approach to designing and providing augmentative and alternative communication (AAC) services for people with a full range of congenital (present at birth) and acquired communication disorders, including those associated with cerebral palsy, autism, aphasia, and traumatic brain injury (TBI). The authors of the chapter focus primarily on the significant number people with of aphasia who experience permanent severe communication disorders. People in this group can sometimes use AAC intervention. Topics include the participation model, communication interaction functions, a communication classification system, assessment considerations, and teaching functional use of AAC strategies. The authors conclude that people with aphasia are increasingly receiving AAC options soon after their strokes. During rehabilitation, therapy to promote the recovery of natural speech is encouraged, and AAC systems are modified to support functional communication that cannot be managed through natural speech. The successful integration of AAC interventions depends also on flexibility and continuity of service delivery as the person with aphasia makes transitions from setting to setting. The chapter includes sidebars that offer relevant quotes from the literature, that share stories from the authors' experiences, and that pose questions for readers to consider while reading the chapter. 11 figures. 2 tables.

- **Assessing Aphasia and Related Disorders**

  Source: in Brookshire, R.H. Introduction to Neurogenic Communication Disorders. 5th ed. St. Louis, MO: Mosby-Year Book, Inc. 1997. p. 127-207.

  Contact: Available from Mosby-Year Book, Inc. 11830 Westline Industrial Drive, P.O. Box 46908, St. Louis, MO 63146. (800) 426-4545; Fax (800) 535-9935; E-mail: customer.support@mosby.com.; http://www.mosby.com. Price: $45.99 plus shipping and handling. ISBN: 0815110146.

  Summary: This chapter on assessing aphasia and related disorders is from a textbook on neurogenic communication disorders. The first section on neuroanatomic explanations of aphasia and related disorders covers language and cerebral dominance, the perisylvian region and language, how the brain performs language, aphasia caused by destruction of the cortical centers for language, aphasia caused by damage to association fiber tracts important to language, and aphasia syndromes without a clear localization. A section of related disorders covers disconnection syndromes, visual field blindness, apraxia, diagnosis of apraxia, apraxia of speech, and agnosia. The next section discusses the assessment of language and communication, including comprehensive language tests, the Minnesota Tests for Differential Diagnosis of Aphasia, the Porch Index of Communicative Ability, he Boston Diagnostic Aphasia Examination, the Western Aphasia Battery, other comprehensive language tests, and screening tests of language and communication. A section on the assessment of auditory comprehension, includes single word comprehension and sentence comprehension, variables that may affect brain-damaged adults' comprehension, sentence comprehension and comprehension in daily life, and comprehension of spoken discourse. Other topics include assessing reading, assessing speech production, assessing written expression, and the effects of managed care on assessment of neurogenic communication disorders. 29 figures. 4 references. (AA-M).

- **Treatment of Aphasia and Related Disorders**

  Source: in Brookshire, R.H. Introduction to Neurogenic Communication Disorders. 5th ed. St. Louis, MO: Mosby-Year Book, Inc. 1997. p. 241-289.

  Contact: Available from Mosby-Year Book, Inc. 11830 Westline Industrial Drive, P.O. Box 46908, St. Louis, MO 63146. (800) 426-4545; Fax (800) 535-9935; E-mail: customer.support@mosby.com.; http://www.mosby.com. Price: $45.99 plus shipping and handling. ISBN: 0815110146.

  Summary: This chapter on the treatment of aphasia and related disorders is from a textbook on neurogenic communication disorders. Sections cover the effectiveness of treatment for aphasia, timing intervention, the goals of treatment, candidacy for treatment, the focus and progression of treatment, treatment of auditory comprehension, treatment of single-word comprehension, understanding spoken sentences, treatment of discourse comprehension, treatment of reading comprehension, treatment of speech production, treating apraxia of speech, writing, and group activities for aphasic adults. Specific topics include answering questions, task switching activities, surface versus deep dyslexia, survival reading skills, readability formulas, commercial reading programs, facilitating volitional speech, behaviors associated with word-retrieval failure, and Melodic Intonation Therapy (MIT). The author notes that some of the principles and procedures presented in this chapter may also apply, in whole or in part, to treatment of communication impairments other than aphasia. 7 figures. 3 tables. (AA-M).

- **Understanding Aphasia**

  Source: in Dilima, S.N.; Niemayer, S., eds. Home Health Care Patient Education Manual. Gaithersburg, MD: Aspen Publishers, Inc. p. 40-41. 1996.

Contact: Available from Aspen Publishers, Inc. 200 Orchard Drive, Gaithersburg, MD 20878. (800) 638-8437; Fax (301) 417-7650. Price: $185.00 plus shipping and handling. Stock Number S124.

Summary: This chapter, from a home health care patient education manual, provides readers with an overview of aphasia. Aphasia is defined as a partial or complete loss of one's ability to speak, gesture, understand spoken words, read, write, or calculate. Topics covered in the chapter include statistics about stroke (the most common cause of aphasia), matching impairment to the affected area of the brain, and the types of impairment. The types of aphasia defined are fluent (receptive) aphasias, nonfluent (expressive) aphasias, and mixed or global aphasias. The author notes that over half of all people who suffer strokes experience speech or language disorders that adversely affect communication.

- **Brain Damage in Aphasia**

Source: in Benson, D.F.; Ardila, A. Aphasia: A Clinical Perspective. New York, NY: Oxford University Press, Inc. 1996. p. 61-87.

Contact: Available from Oxford University Press, Inc. 200 Madison Avenue, New York, NY 10016. (800) 334-4249 or (212) 679-7300. Price: $49.95 plus shipping and handling. ISBN: 0195089340.

Summary: This chapter on brain damage in aphasia is from a book that presents an integrated analysis of the language disturbances associated with brain pathology. The authors note that the underlying disease process must be recognized and treated along with the language problem; both the type of language therapy offered and the patient's prognosis depend on the basic pathology. The authors discuss some of the more common brain disorders associated with aphasia, including vascular disorders (thrombosis, embolism, hemorrhage), trauma, intracranial neoplasms, infections (including intracranial abscess), and miscellaneous causes of aphasia, including multiple sclerosis, epilepsy, Alzheimer's disease, Jakob-Creutzfeldt disease, and progressive aphasia. The authors continue by discussing localization techniques (to locate the neuroanatomical site of brain damage in cases of aphasia), neuropathology, neurosurgery, posttrauma skull defects, the neurologic examination, and brain-imaging studies. The authors conclude that the localization of aphasia-producing lesions has advanced tremendously in the past several decades, particularly with the advent of noninvasive techniques that can produce accurate anatomical localizations. 10 figures. 2 tables. (AA-M).

- **Management and Rehabilitation of Aphasia**

  Source: in Benson, D.F.; Ardila, A. Aphasia: A Clinical Perspective. New York, NY: Oxford University Press, Inc. 1996. p. 354-364.

  Contact: Available from Oxford University Press, Inc. 200 Madison Avenue, New York, NY 10016. (800) 334-4249 or (212) 679-7300. Price: $49.95 plus shipping and handling. ISBN: 0195089340.

  Summary: This chapter on the management and rehabilitation of aphasia is from a book that presents an integrated analysis of the language disturbances associated with brain pathology. The authors utilize an analogy of living in a foreign-language environment to help readers comprehend the techniques of simple grammar, clear pronunciation, and redundancy when working with patients with aphasia. Topics covered include language rehabilitation, basic factors, the effectiveness of aphasia therapy, long-term considerations, aphasia therapy methodology, the stimulus-facilitation technique, programmed learning techniques, deblocking, functional system reorganization, melodic intonation therapy (MIT), sign language, visual symbol communication systems, and computers in aphasia rehabilitation. The authors conclude that at present, specific, problem-directed therapy is available for only a few language deficits and their use is not imperative. MIT, the best-known and most rigidly exact language therapy technique, has proved effective for only a limited and strictly designated group of aphasic patients. (AA-M).

- **Landau-Kleffner Syndrome (Acquired Epileptic Aphasia)**

  Source: in DeFeo, A.B., ed. Parent Articles 2. San Antonio, TX: Communication Skill Builders. 1995. p. 151-152.

  Contact: Available from Communication Skill Builders. Customer Service, 555 Academic Court, San Antonio, TX 78204-2498. (800) 211-8378; Fax (800) 232-1223. Price: $55.00 plus shipping and handling. Order Number 076-163-0732.

  Summary: This fact sheet, from a communication skills book for parents, provides information on Landau-Kleffner syndrome (acquired epileptic aphasia). Topics covered include the incidence of Landau-Kleffner, the medical aspects of the disorder, language aspects of Landau-Kleffner, testing and assessment issues, and tips for promoting language development. The author provides detailed suggestions for parent-child interaction, including recommended activities. The author encourages parents to incorporate these suggestions into everyday routines and to act as their child's advocate. 1 reference.

- **Landau-Kleffner Syndrome (Acquired Epileptic Aphasia)**

  Source: in DeFeo, A.B., ed. Parent Articles 2. San Antonio, TX: Communication Skill Builders. 1995. p. 151-152.

  Contact: Available from Communication Skill Builders. Customer Service, 555 Academic Court, San Antonio, TX 78204-2498. (800) 211-8378; Fax (800) 232-1223. Price: $55.00 plus shipping and handling. Order Number 076-163-0732.

  Summary: This fact sheet, from a communication skills book for parents, provides information on Landau-Kleffner syndrome (acquired epileptic aphasia). Topics covered include the incidence of Landau-Kleffner, the medical aspects of the disorder, language aspects of Landau-Kleffner, testing and assessment issues, and tips for promoting language development. The author provides detailed suggestions for parent-child interaction, including recommended activities. The author encourages parents to incorporate these suggestions into everyday routines and to act as their child's advocate. 1 reference.

Directories

In addition to the references and resources discussed earlier in this chapter, a number of directories relating to aphasia have been published that consolidate information across various sources. These too might be useful in gaining access to additional guidance on aphasia. The Combined Health Information Database lists the following, which you may wish to consult in your local medical library:[24]

- **Brain Connections: Your Source Guide to Information on Brain Diseases and Disorders. 5th ed**

  Source: New York, NY: Dana Alliance for Brain Initiatives. 2000. 49 p.

  Contact: Available from Dana Press. Charles A. Dana Foundation, 745 Fifth Avenue, Suite 700, New York, NY 10151. Fax (212) 593-7623. Website: www.dana.org. PRICE: Single copy free.

---

[24] You will need to limit your search to "Directories" and aphasia using the "Detailed Search" option. Go directly to the following hyperlink: **http://chid.nih.gov/detail/detail.html**. To find directories, use the drop boxes at the bottom of the search page where "You may refine your search by". For publication date, select "All Years", select language and the format option "Directory". By making these selections and typing in "aphasia" (or synonyms) into the "For these words:" box, you will only receive results on directories dealing with aphasia. You should check back periodically with this database as it is updated every three months.

Summary: This guide lists organizations that assist people with a brain-related disorder or disease as well as those organizations that assist caregivers and health care providers in these areas. The guide lists more than 275 organizations alphabetically by disease or disorder. Listings of particular relevance to communication disorders include: acoustic neuroma, aphasia, ataxia, attention deficit hyperactivity disorder, autism, deafness and hearing loss, disability and rehabilitation, dizziness, dyslexia, dystonia, head injury, learning disabilities, neurofibromatosis, smell and taste (chemosensory) disorders, spasmodic dysphonia, stuttering, tinnitus, Tourette syndrome, and vestibular disorders. Emphasis is placed on organizations that have a national focus, however, many of these groups sponsor local chapters or affiliates and make referrals to local medical professionals and organizations. For each organization listed, the guide notes mailing address, telephone numbers, e-mail and web sites; also provided are symbols which indicate that the organization offers support groups, referrals to doctors, referrals to other sources of information, regional chapters, availability of literature, availability of speakers, and volunteer opportunities. The guide also describes the publishing body, the Dana Alliance for Brain Initiatives, and provides a list of ways in which readers can support and further brain research.

- **Aphasia Community Groups**

Source: New York, NY: National Aphasia Association. 1997. 21 p.

Contact: National Aphasia Association. Distribution Center, 351 Butternut Court, Millersville, MD 21108. (800) 922-4622; http://www.aphasia.org. PRICE: $2.50 each.

Summary: This directory lists aphasia community groups. Some groups consist only of persons with aphasia and their significant others. Other groups may be more inclusive and may include other family members, friends, and professionals. Some of the groups are free of charge. The most recent listing for each individual group can be accessed by calling 1-800-922-4NAA. The listing is organized alphabetically by state; a few Canadian groups are also included. The directory concludes with a brief list of resource organizations that might have additional information about groups. (AA-M).

- **Associations and Agencies**

Source: New York, NY: National Aphasia Association. 1997. 2 p.

Contact: National Aphasia Association. Distribution Center, 351 Butternut Court, Millersville, MD 21108. (800) 922-4622; http://www.aphasia.org. PRICE: $0.25 each.

Summary: This fact sheet, written for the general public, provides a listing of associations and agencies for obtaining additional information on aphasia. The directory lists organizations alphabetically by name of the organization. Each entry includes an address and telephone number; some entries include one sentence that briefly describes the information or services available. For example, the National Stroke Association offers several free and low cost publications of interest to persons with aphasia and their families. Seventeen organizations are listed.

- **NAA Regional and Area Representatives**

  Source: New York, NY: National Aphasia Association. 1997. 7 p.

  Contact: Available from National Aphasia Association. 156 Fifth Avenue, Suite 707, New York, NY 10010. (800) 922-4662 or (212) 255-4329; http://www.aphasia.org. PRICE: $1 plus $3 shipping; also available with information packet on aphasia (for a donation).

  Summary: This fact sheet lists regional and area representatives of the National Aphasia Association (NAA). These representatives are health care professionals who have volunteered to receive calls from families. They can help callers become acquainted with local resources for persons with aphasia. The United States is divided into 14 regions. The list provides the addresses and telephone numbers for the representatives in each region.

General Home References

In addition to references for aphasia, you may want a general home medical guide that spans all aspects of home healthcare. The following list is a recent sample of such guides (sorted alphabetically by title; hyperlinks provide rankings, information, and reviews at Amazon.com):

- **Human Communication Disorders: An Introduction** by George H. Shames, et al; Hardcover - 768 pages, 5th edition (February 3, 1998), Allyn & Bacon; ISBN: 0205270026; **http://www.amazon.com/exec/obidos/ASIN/0205270026/icongroupinterna**

- **Management of Motor Speech Disorders in Children and Adults** by Kathryn M. Yorkston (Editor); Hardcover, 2nd edition (July 2001), Pro Ed;

ISBN: 0890797846;
http://www.amazon.com/exec/obidos/ASIN/0890797846/icongroupinterna

Vocabulary Builder

Ataxia: Failure of muscular coordination; irregularity of muscular action. [EU]

Atypical: Irregular; not conformable to the type; in microbiology, applied specifically to strains of unusual type. [EU]

Blindness: The inability to see or the loss or absence of perception of visual stimuli. This condition may be the result of eye diseases; optic nerve diseases; optic chiasm diseases; or brain diseases affecting the visual pathways or occipital lobe. [NIH]

Conduction: The transfer of sound waves, heat, nervous impulses, or electricity. [EU]

Dizziness: An imprecise term which may refer to a sense of spatial disorientation, motion of the environment, or lightheadedness. [NIH]

Dominance: In genetics, the full phenotypic expression of a gene in both heterozygotes and homozygotes. [EU]

Dystonia: Disordered tonicity of muscle. [EU]

Hemorrhage: Bleeding or escape of blood from a vessel. [NIH]

Neoplasms: New abnormal growth of tissue. Malignant neoplasms show a greater degree of anaplasia and have the properties of invasion and metastasis, compared to benign neoplasms. [NIH]

Neuropsychology: A branch of psychology which investigates the correlation between experience or behavior and the basic neurophysiological processes. The term neuropsychology stresses the dominant role of the nervous system. It is a more narrowly defined field than physiological psychology or psychophysiology. [NIH]

Neurosurgery: A surgical specialty concerned with the treatment of diseases and disorders of the brain, spinal cord, and peripheral and sympathetic nervous system. [NIH]

Phonation: The process of producing vocal sounds by means of vocal cords vibrating in an expiratory blast of air. [NIH]

Skull: The skeleton of the head including the bones of the face and the bones enclosing the brain. [NIH]

Thrombosis: The formation, development, or presence of a thrombus. [EU]

Tinnitus: A noise in the ears, as ringing, buzzing, roaring, clicking, etc. Such sounds may at times be heard by others than the patient. [EU]

Vestibular: Pertaining to or toward a vestibule. In dental anatomy, used to refer to the tooth surface directed toward the vestibule of the mouth. [EU]

CHAPTER 6. MULTIMEDIA ON APHASIA

Overview

Information on aphasia can come in a variety of formats. Among multimedia sources, video productions, slides, audiotapes, and computer databases are often available. In this chapter, we show you how to keep current on multimedia sources of information on aphasia. We start with sources that have been summarized by federal agencies, and then show you how to find bibliographic information catalogued by the National Library of Medicine. If you see an interesting item, visit your local medical library to check on the availability of the title.

Video Recordings

Most diseases do not have a video dedicated to them. If they do, they are often rather technical in nature. An excellent source of multimedia information on aphasia is the Combined Health Information Database. You will need to limit your search to "video recording" and "aphasia" using the "Detailed Search" option. Go directly to the following hyperlink: **http://chid.nih.gov/detail/detail.html**. To find video productions, use the drop boxes at the bottom of the search page where "You may refine your search by." Select the dates and language you prefer, and the format option "Videorecording (videotape, videocassette, etc.)." By making these selections and typing "aphasia" (or synonyms) into the "For these words:" box, you will only receive results on video productions. The following is a typical result when searching for video recordings on aphasia:

- **Pathways: Moving Beyond Stroke and Aphasia**

   Source: Detroit, MI: Wayne State University Press. 1991.

Contact: Available from Wayne State University Press. Leonard N. Simons Building, 5959 Woodward Avenue, Detroit, MI 48201-6131. (800) 978-7323 or (313) 577-6120; Fax (313) 577-6131. PRICE: $49.95 plus shipping and handling.

Summary: With the assistance of six individuals and their families, this videotape is designed to encourage and motivate stroke survivors and their families in the recovery stages of stroke and rehabilitation so that they too can, in time, move beyond their illness (AA).

- **Aphasia and Augmentative Communication: Strategies for Increasing Participation in Life Activities**

  Source: Tucson, AZ: National Center for Neurogenic Communication Disorders, University of Arizona. 2000. (videocassette).

  Contact: Available from National Center for Neurogenic Communication Disorders, University of Arizona. P.O. Box 210071, Tucson, AZ 85721-0071. (520) 621-1472. Fax (520) 621-2226. PRICE: $25.00 plus shipping and handling. Order Number TR-54.

  Summary: This videotape program, which is part of the Telerounds videoconference series from the National Center for Neurogenic Communication Disorders at the University of Arizona (funded partly by NIDCD), is the third teleconference in a three part series on augmentative and alternative communication (AAC). The speaker introduces the viewer to principles of using AAC with people who have aphasia. This acquired disorder impacts receptive and expressive language. The principles of using AAC strategies include helping people with aphasia participate in meaningful adult activities, matching the AAC strategy to the cognitive and linguistic skills of the communicator, and providing learning during contextualized and interactive communication. The speaker discusses the challenges of using AAC with people who have aphasia and presents considerations for selecting and incorporating AAC strategies into an overall communication package. In addition, the speaker describes and illustrates controlled context, augmented input, and comprehensive communicators using videotaped segments. Instructional techniques are also briefly reviewed, including role playing, scripting, and trials with alternative communication partners. The program concludes by answering questions asked by the host and phoned in by the teleconference audience and by providing information about joining Centernet, the online forum operated by the Center.

- **Computer Applications in Aphasia Rehabilitation**

  Source: Tucson, AZ: National Center for Neurogenic Communication Disorders, University of Arizona. 1997. (videocassette).

  Contact: National Center for Neurogenic Communication Disorders, University of Arizona. P.O. Box 210071, Tucson, AZ 85721-0071. (521) 621-1472. Fax (520) 621-2226. PRICE: $40.00. Order number TR-38.

  Summary: This videocassette program is one in a series of Telerounds Continuing Education from the National Center for Neurogenic Communication Disorders at the University of Arizona (funded partly by NIDCD). This program describes research in the uses of computers in speech pathology (particularly aphasia). One presenter reviews changes in computer applications and relevant literature and concludes that computers can be beneficial, but require considerable input from clinicians. While computers fall short of replacing clinicians, they can be very useful as part of speech language therapy. Simulations (microworlds) are helpful, and are more effective than drill-and-practice type tasks. The program shows a clinician working with a patient on the computer. The program concludes by answering questions phoned in by the teleconference audience and by providing information about joining Centernet, the online forum run by the Center.

- **Chronic Broca's Aphasia: Evidence for Right Hemisphere Language**

  Source: Tucson, AZ: National Center for Neurogenic Communication Disorders. 1995. (videocassette and handout).

  Contact: Available from National Center for Neurogenic Communication Disorders. Telerounds Coordinator, Building 71, Room 500, University of Arizona, Tucson, AZ 85721. (520) 621-1819 or (520) 621-1472. PRICE: $25.00.

  Summary: The question regarding what anatomical structures mediate the residual language functions of individuals with chronic Broca's aphasia has been of long-standing interest. In this telerounds program, the authors describe two right-handed males who experienced massive strokes that caused extensive destruction of the left hemisphere, resulting in classic Broca's aphasia. They discuss how these individuals' language performance is consistent with right hemisphere language capacity, and conclude that Broca's aphasia can result when language is mediated exclusively by the nondominant hemisphere. The handout provided with the videotape includes an abstract, a list of objectives, a brief outline of the program, a reference list, and an evaluation form for viewers to complete and return. (AA-M).

- **Pragmatics, Syntax and Aphasia**

  Source: Tucson, AZ: National Center for Neurogenic Communication Disorders, University of Arizona. November 29, 1995. (videocassette and handout).

  Contact: Available from National Center for Neurogenic Communication Disorders. University of Arizona, P.O. Box 210071, Tucson, AZ 85721-0071. (602) 621-1819 or (602) 621-1787. PRICE: $25.00 plus shipping and handling.

  Summary: This program provides an overview of the pragmatic aspects of language, i.e., the ways that choosing different words and grammatical constructions are appropriate for different communicative goals. Most areas of pragmatics are relatively spared in aphasia; these are contrasted with the few that are impaired. The program shows how preserved pragmatics can interact with impaired syntax to produce utterances which are the opposite of what the person with aphasia means to say. The program provides suggestions for how the patient can learn to monitor for and avoid these semantically 'reversed' utterances. 10 references. (AA).

- **Aphasia Groups: An Approach to Long-Term Rehabilitation**

  Source: Tucson, AZ: National Center for Neurogenic Communication Disorders. 1994. (videocassette and handout).

  Contact: Available from National Center for Neurogenic Communication Disorders. Telerounds Coordinator, Building 71, Room 500, University of Arizona, Tucson, AZ 85721. (520) 621-1819 or (520) 621-1472. PRICE: $25.00.

  Summary: This telerounds program is designed to demonstrate how various aphasia group sessions might be structured to achieve the goals of maximizing communication effectiveness and lessening the negative impact of aphasia on the lives of the group members. The program notes that there is increasing interest in the group format as a means of addressing the disability caused by the aphasia, as well as a response to health care cost containment. The panel reports on 3 years of experience with small group formats at the University of Arizona. The handout provided with the videotape includes an abstract, a list of objectives, a brief outline of the program, a reference list, and an evaluation form for viewers to complete and return. (AA-M).

- **Progressive Aphasia: An Overview and Case in Point**

  Source: Tucson, AZ: National Center for Neurogenic Communication Disorders. 1994. (videocassette and handout).

  Contact: Available from National Center for Neurogenic Communication Disorders. Telerounds Coordinator, Building 71, Room 500, University of Arizona, Tucson, AZ 85721. (520) 621-1819 or (520) 621-1472. PRICE: $25.00.

  Summary: This telerounds program provides an overview of progressive aphasia and presents a case study of an individual with this disorder. Topics covered include a definition of progressive aphasia; the results of longitudinal investigations of patients with progressive aphasia; the interplay of aphasia and Alzheimer's disease; and the neuropathological changes associated with progressive aphasia. The handout provided with the videotape includes an abstract, a list of objectives, a brief outline of the program, a reference list, and an evaluation form for viewers to complete and return. The handout also includes the details of the case study presented, as well as a chart summarizes numerous related cases presented in the literature. 33 references. (AA-M).

- **Cerebral Localization of Production Deficits in Aphasia**

  Source: Tucson, AZ: National Center for Neurogenic Communication Disorders, University of Arizona. March 31, 1993. (videocassette and handout).

  Contact: Available from National Center for Neurogenic Communication Disorders. University of Arizona, P.O. Box 210071, Tucson, AZ 85721-0071. (602) 621-1819 or (602) 621-1787. PRICE: $25.00 plus shipping and handling.

  Summary: This videotape program discusses a new method of evaluating the relationship between lesion site and specific speech and language disorders. Three new findings with regard to the neuroanatomic correlates of non-fluent production problems in aphasia are introduced. First, the consistent relationship between apraxia of speech and a particular area of the insula is presented. Next, the involvement of the arcuate fasciculus is discussed in conjunction with the severe production problems characterized by recurring utterances. Finally, the possibility that the angular gyrus might be involved in agrammatic behavior is explored. 26 references. (AA).

- **Mining for Gold: Identifying Preserved Abilities in Severe Aphasia**

  Source: Tucson, AZ: National Center for Neurogenic Communication Disorders, University of Arizona. 1992. (videocassette and handout).

  Contact: National Center for Neurogenic Communication Disorders. University of Arizona, P.O. Box 210071, Tucson, AZ 85721-0071. (602) 621-1819 or (602) 621-1787. Price: $25.00 plus shipping and handling.

  Summary: This videotape program is one in a series of video-conferences, called Telerounds, designed for speech-language pathologists and allied health care professionals. Telerounds, a continuing education program, is supported by the University of Arizona National Center for Neurogenic Communication Disorders. This video teleconference focuses on the problems of assessing and treating patients with forms of severe aphasia. Techniques for identifying preserved abilities and maximizing performance in severe aphasia are explored with two patients, one with severe nonfluent (but not global) aphasia and one with severe fluent (but not Wernicke's) aphasia. Possible applications of the results to treatment are discussed. A booklet accompanying the video describes the objectives and contents of the videotape. The booklet includes an evaluation form for the teleconference. A list of suggested readings is provided. 4 references. (AA-M).

- **What is Aphasia?**

  Source: Detroit, MI: Wayne State University Press. 1991.

  Contact: Available from Wayne State University Press. Leonard N. Simons Building, 5959 Woodward Avenue, Detroit, MI 48201-6131. (800) 978-7323 or (313) 577-6120; Fax (313) 577-6131. PRICE: $49.95 plus shipping and handling.

  Summary: This videotape is for patients and families. Stroke survivors demonstrate their strategies to compensate for communication losses, while family members share experiences of learning to communicate effectively with aphasic individuals. Examples and analogies explain aphasia and its effects on speaking, listening, reading, and writing (AA-M).

Bibliography: Multimedia on Aphasia

The National Library of Medicine is a rich source of information on healthcare-related multimedia productions including slides, computer software, and databases. To access the multimedia database, go to the following Web site: **http://locatorplus.gov/**. Select "Search LOCATORplus." Once in the search area, simply type in aphasia (or synonyms). Then, in the option box provided below the search box, select "Audiovisuals and Computer Files." From there, you can choose to sort results by publication date, author, or relevance. The following multimedia has been indexed on aphasia. For more information, follow the hyperlink indicated:

- **Aphasia and augmentative communication : strategies for increasing participation in life activities.** Source: produced by the National Center for Neurogenic Communication Disorders of the University of Arizona; Year: 2000; Format: Videorecording; Tucson, AZ: Arizona Board of Regents, c2000

- **Aphasia groups : an approach to long-term rehabilitation.** Source: the National Center for Neurogenic Communication Disorders; [with the cooperation of] Veterans Health Administration, Office of Academic Affairs [and] Long Beach Regional Medical; Year: 1994; Format: Videorecording; [Tucson, Ariz.]: Arizona Board of Regents, c1994

- **Aphasic agrammatism : underlying causes and overt manifestations.** Source: the National Center for Neurogenic Communication Disorders; the National Institute on Deafness and Other Communication Disorders; Veterans Health Administration, Office; Year: 1993; Format: Videorecording; [Tucson, Ariz.]: Arizona Board of Regents, c1993

- **Baker's clinical neurology on CD-ROM.** Source: Robert J. Joynt, Robert C. Griggs; Year: 2000; Format: Electronic resource; [Baltimore?]: Lippincott Williams & Wilkins, c2000

- **Case of aphasia : showing difficulty in word-finding, in comprehension, and in handling complex ideas.** Source: from the Henry Phipps Psychiatric Clinic and Spring Grove State Hospital of Maryland; Year: 1939; Format: Motion picture; [United States]: Psychological Cinema Register of the Pennsylvania State College, 1939

- **Cerebral localization of production deficits in aphasia.** Source: [produced by] the National Center for Neurogenic Communication Disorders; Year: 1993; Format: Videorecording; [Tucson]: Arizona Board of Regents, c1993

- **Chronic Broca's aphasia : evidence for right hemisphere language.** Source: produced by the National Center for Neurogenic Communication Disorders of the University of Arizona; Year: 1995; Format: Videorecording; Tucson, Ariz.: Arizona Board of Regents, c1995

- **Co-constructing meaning in conversations with a man with severe aphasia.** Source: produced by the National Center for Neurogenic Communication Disorders of the University of Arizona; Year: 1996; Format: Videorecording; [Tucson, Ariz.]: Arizona Board of Regents, c1996

- **Communicating with the aphasic patient.** Source: produced by Fairview General Hospital; Year: 1982; Format: Videorecording; Cleveland, Ohio: The Hospital, c1982

- **Computer applications in aphasia rehabilitation.** Source: produced by the National Center for Neurogenic Communication Disorders of the University of Arizona; Year: 1997; Format: Videorecording; Tucson, Ariz.: Arizona Board of Regents, c1997

- **Diagnosing and treating aphasia : Alexander Luria's systems approach to brain behavior relationships.** Source: video production by Studio 6 Productions; Year: 1991; Format: Videorecording; Orlando, FL: Paul M. Deutsch Press, c1991

- **Examining for aphasia with the Boston Diagnostic Aphasia Examination (third edition).** Source: Harold Goodglass with the collaboration of Edith Kaplan and Barbara Barresi; Year: 2001; Format: Videorecording; Hagerstown, MD: Lippincott Williams & Wilkins, c2001

- **Help me, reach me : alterations in communication: aphasia.** Source: University of Wisconsin-Milwaukee, School of Nursing; a Television Services production, University of Wisconsin-Milwaukee; Year: 1985; Format: Videorecording; [Philadelphia, Pa.]: Lippincott, c1985

- **How to communicate with someone who has aphasia.** Source: a Healing Arts Communications [and] Media Works production; Year: 2000; Format: Videorecording; Syracuse, NY: Program Development Associates, c2000

- **Inner world of aphasia.** Source: Leonard Pearson; produced by Edward Feil Productions; Year: 1968; Format: Motion picture; Cleveland, Ohio: Pearson: [for loan and sale by Feil Productions; Atlanta: for loan by National Medical Audiovisual Center, 1968]

- **Introduction to aphasia.** Source: Dept. of Medicine and Surgery, Veterans Administration; [made by] Churchill Wexler; Year: 1950; Format: Motion picture; [Chicago]: American Medical Assn., 1950

- **Language disorders (aphasia).** Source: Concept Media [in cooperation with] Dept. of Medical Education, Memorial Hospital of Long Beach; Year: 1969; Format: Filmstrip; [Costa Mesa, Calif.]: Concept Media, c1969

- **Mining for gold : identifying preserved abilities in severe aphasia.** Source: the National Center for Neurogenic Communication Disorders; the National Institute on Deafness and Other Communication Disorders; Veterans Administration,Office of Ac; Year: 1992; Format: Videorecording; [Tucson, Ariz.]: Arizona Board of Regents, c1992

- **Pragmatics, syntax, and aphasia.** Source: produced by the National Center for Neurogenic Communication Disorders of the University of

Arizona; Year: 1995; Format: Videorecording; [Tucson, Ariz.]: Arizona Board of Regents, c1995

- **Primary progressive aphasia.** Source: produced by the National Center for Neurogenic Communication Disorders of the University of Arizona; Year: 1996; Format: Videorecording; [Tucson, Ariz.]: Arizona Board of Regents, c1996

- **Progressive aphasia : overview and case in point.** Source: [presented by] the National Center for Neurogenic Communication Disorders; Veterans Health Administration, Office of Academic Affairs, Long Beach Regional Medical Education Center; Year: 1993; Format: Videorecording; Tucson, Ariz.: Arizona Board of Regents, c1993

- **Speech and hearing changes in aging.** Source: presented by Center for the Study of Aging, in cooperation with the Health Communications Network, and the Geriatric Education Center, University of Alabama at Birmingham; Year: 1991; Format: Videorecording; Charleston, S.C.: Medical University of South Carolina, c1991

- **Stroke : focus on apraxia and aphasia.** Source: an AREN production; [produced at the facilities of WQED/Pittsburgh by QED Enterprises]; Year: 1986; Format: Videorecording; [Pittsburgh, Pa.]: AREN, c1986

- **Therapeutic communication : dementia & aphasia.** Source: Beacon Health Corporation; Year: 1991; Format: Videorecording; Mequon, WI: The Corporation, c1991

- **Verbal impairment associated with brain damage.** Source: Institute of Physical Medicine and Rehabilitation, New York University Medical Center; produced by Public Health Service Audiovisual Facility; Year: 1966; Format: Motion picture; Atlanta: National Medical Audiovisual Center; [Washington: for sale by National Audiovisual Center, 1966]

CHAPTER 7. PERIODICALS AND NEWS ON APHASIA

Overview

Keeping up on the news relating to aphasia can be challenging. Subscribing to targeted periodicals can be an effective way to stay abreast of recent developments on aphasia. Periodicals include newsletters, magazines, and academic journals.

In this chapter, we suggest a number of news sources and present various periodicals that cover aphasia beyond and including those which are published by patient associations mentioned earlier. We will first focus on news services, and then on periodicals. News services, press releases, and newsletters generally use more accessible language, so if you do chose to subscribe to one of the more technical periodicals, make sure that it uses language you can easily follow.

News Services & Press Releases

Well before articles show up in newsletters or the popular press, they may appear in the form of a press release or a public relations announcement. One of the simplest ways of tracking press releases on aphasia is to search the news wires. News wires are used by professional journalists, and have existed since the invention of the telegraph. Today, there are several major "wires" that are used by companies, universities, and other organizations to announce new medical breakthroughs. In the following sample of sources, we will briefly describe how to access each service. These services only post recent news intended for public viewing.

PR Newswire

Perhaps the broadest of the wires is PR Newswire Association, Inc. To access this archive, simply go to **http://www.prnewswire.com**. Below the search box, select the option "The last 30 days." In the search box, type "aphasia" or synonyms. The search results are shown by order of relevance. When reading these press releases, do not forget that the sponsor of the release may be a company or organization that is trying to sell a particular product or therapy. Their views, therefore, may be biased.

Reuters

The Reuters' Medical News database can be very useful in exploring news archives relating to aphasia. While some of the listed articles are free to view, others can be purchased for a nominal fee. To access this archive, go to **http://www.reutershealth.com/frame2/arch.html** and search by "aphasia" (or synonyms). The following was recently listed in this archive for aphasia:

- **Dextroamphetamine speeds recovery from aphasia in stroke patients**
  Source: Reuters Industry Breifing
  Date: September 07, 2001
  http://www.reuters.gov/archive/2001/09/07/business/links/20010907clin004.html

- **Recovery from aphasia due to left-lobe stroke lesion linked to activation of other areas**
  Source: Reuters Medical News
  Date: December 25, 2000
  http://www.reuters.gov/archive/2000/12/25/professional/links/20001225scie003.html

- **Site of infarct predicts recovery from poststroke aphasia**
  Source: Reuters Medical News
  Date: October 23, 1998
  http://www.reuters.gov/archive/1998/10/23/professional/links/19981023clin012.html

- **Stroke-related aphasia modifiable when interventions targeted at unaffected hemisphere**
  Source: Reuters Medical News
  Date: June 05, 1998
  http://www.reuters.gov/archive/1998/06/05/professional/links/19980605clin010.html

- **AAN Report: Poststroke Aphasia Recovery Poorer With Right Hemispheric Activation**
  Source: Reuters Medical News
  Date: May 01, 1998
  http://www.reuters.gov/archive/1998/05/01/professional/links/19980501scie001.html

The NIH

Within MEDLINEplus, the NIH has made an agreement with the New York Times Syndicate, the AP News Service, and Reuters to deliver news that can be browsed by the public. Search news releases at **http://www.nlm.nih.gov/medlineplus/alphanews_a.html.** MEDLINEplus allows you to browse across an alphabetical index. Or you can search by date at **http://www.nlm.nih.gov/medlineplus/newsbydate.html**. Often, news items are indexed by MEDLINEplus within their search engine.

Business Wire

Business Wire is similar to PR Newswire. To access this archive, simply go to **http://www.businesswire.com**. You can scan the news by industry category or company name.

Internet Wire

Internet Wire is more focused on technology than the other wires. To access this site, go to **http://www.internetwire.com** and use the "Search Archive" option. Type in "aphasia" (or synonyms). As this service is oriented to technology, you may wish to search for press releases covering diagnostic procedures or tests that you may have read about.

Search Engines

Free-to-view news can also be found in the news section of your favorite search engines (see the health news page at Yahoo: **http://dir.yahoo.com/Health/News_and_Media/,** or use this Web site's general news search page **http://news.yahoo.com/.** Type in "aphasia" (or synonyms). If you know the name of a company that is relevant to aphasia, you can go to any stock trading Web site (such as **www.etrade.com**) and search for the company name there. News items across various news sources are reported on indicated hyperlinks.

BBC

Covering news from a more European perspective, the British Broadcasting Corporation (BBC) allows the public free access to their news archive located at **http://www.bbc.co.uk/**. Search by "aphasia" (or synonyms).

Newsletter Articles

If you choose not to subscribe to a newsletter, you can nevertheless find references to newsletter articles. We recommend that you use the Combined Health Information Database, while limiting your search criteria to "newsletter articles." Again, you will need to use the "Detailed Search" option. Go to the following hyperlink: **http://chid.nih.gov/detail/detail.html**. Go to the bottom of the search page where "You may refine your search by." Select the dates and language that you prefer. For the format option, select "Newsletter Article."

By making these selections, and typing in "aphasia" (or synonyms) into the "For these words:" box, you will only receive results on newsletter articles. You should check back periodically with this database as it is updated every 3 months. The following is a typical result when searching for newsletter articles on aphasia:

- **Speech After Stroke: Rehabilitation Enhances Recovery and Lifestyle**

  Source: Mayo Clinic Health Letter. 14(8): 1-3. August 1996.

  Contact: Available from Mayo Foundation for Medical Education and Research. 200 First Street, S.W., Rochester, MN 55905. (800) 633-4567. PRICE: $3.00 for single copy of newsletter plus shipping and handling.

  Summary: This newsletter article describes advances in post-stroke speech and language rehabilitation. Topics include how stroke damages brain cells; the three main stroke-related communication disorders, aphasia, dysarthria, and apraxia; how speech rehabilitation can enhance quality of life for people who have had a stroke; diagnosing speech and language problems; the components of a speech rehabilitation program, including exercise and practice, and the use of picture cards, picture boards, workbooks, and computers; and the psychosocial impact of recovering from a stroke. One sidebar outlines the role of family and friends in the recovery process.

- **Landau-Kleffner Syndrome**

  Source: T.A.L.K. Taking Action Against Language Disorders in Kids. 3(3): 2-7. Fall 1994.

  Contact: Available from Taking Action Against Language Disorders in Kids (TALK). 22980 Donna Lane, Bend, OR 97701. (503) 389-0004.

  Summary: This newsletter article focuses on Landau-Kleffner Syndrome (LKS), a rare condition in which children first lose the ability to understand others, and then lose their ability to speak. The abilities of children with LKS may fluctuate, with periods of remission followed by deterioration. While losing the ability to speak, they can often read and write, and can learn sign language. This article describes the symptoms of LKS and then discusses behavioral problems; the similarities betweeb LKS and autism; hearing tests and other diagnostic tests used; the etiology of LKS; and a comparison of LKS to aphasia. An accompanying article, reprinted from the Philadelphia Enquirer newspaper, describes one family's experiences with LKS in their child.

Academic Periodicals covering Aphasia

Academic periodicals can be a highly technical yet valuable source of information on aphasia. We have compiled the following list of periodicals known to publish articles relating to aphasia and which are currently indexed within the National Library of Medicine's PubMed database (follow hyperlinks to view more information, summaries, etc., for each). In addition to these sources, to keep current on articles written on aphasia published by any of the periodicals listed below, you can simply follow the hyperlink indicated or go to the following Web site: **www.ncbi.nlm.nih.gov/pubmed**. Type the periodical's name into the search box to find the latest studies published.

If you want complete details about the historical contents of a periodical, you can also visit **http://www.ncbi.nlm.nih.gov/entrez/jrbrowser.cgi**. Here, type in the name of the journal or its abbreviation, and you will receive an index of published articles. At **http://locatorplus.gov/** you can retrieve more indexing information on medical periodicals (e.g. the name of the publisher). Select the button "Search LOCATORplus." Then type in the name of the journal and select the advanced search option "Journal Title Search." The following is a sample of periodicals which publish articles on aphasia:

- **Archives of Physical Medicine and Rehabilitation. (Arch Phys Med Rehabil)**
  http://www.ncbi.nlm.nih.gov/entrez/jrbrowser.cgi?field=0&regexp=Archives+of+Physical+Medicine+and+Rehabilitation&dispmax=20&dispstart=0

- **British Journal of Nursing (Mark Allen Publishing). (Br J Nurs)**
  http://www.ncbi.nlm.nih.gov/entrez/jrbrowser.cgi?field=0&regexp=British+Journal+of+Nursing+(Mark+Allen+Publishing)&dispmax=20&dispstart=0

- **Disability and Rehabilitation. (Disabil Rehabil)**
  http://www.ncbi.nlm.nih.gov/entrez/jrbrowser.cgi?field=0&regexp=Disability+and+Rehabilitation&dispmax=20&dispstart=0

- **International Journal of Language & Communication Disorders / Royal College of Speech & Language Therapists. (Int J Lang Commun Disord)**
  http://www.ncbi.nlm.nih.gov/entrez/jrbrowser.cgi?field=0&regexp=International+Journal+of+Language+&+Communication+Disorders+/+Royal+College+of+Speech+&+Language+Therapists&dispmax=20&dispstart=0

- **International Journal of Rehabilitation Research. Internationale Zeitschrift Fur Rehabilitationsforschung. Revue Internationale De Recherches De Readaptation. (Int J Rehabil Res)**
  http://www.ncbi.nlm.nih.gov/entrez/jrbrowser.cgi?field=0&regexp=International+Journal+of+Rehabilitation+Research.+Internationale+Zeitschrift+Fur+Rehabilitationsforschung.+Revue+Internationale+De+Recherches+De+Readaptation&dispmax=20&dispstart=0

- **Journal of Communication Disorders. (J Commun Disord)**
  http://www.ncbi.nlm.nih.gov/entrez/jrbrowser.cgi?field=0&regexp=Journal+of+Communication+Disorders&dispmax=20&dispstart=0

- **Journal of Speech and Hearing Research. (J Speech Hear Res)**
  http://www.ncbi.nlm.nih.gov/entrez/jrbrowser.cgi?field=0&regexp=Journal+of+Speech+and+Hearing+Research&dispmax=20&dispstart=0

- **Journal of Speech, Language, and Hearing Research : Jslhr. (J Speech Lang Hear Res)**
  http://www.ncbi.nlm.nih.gov/entrez/jrbrowser.cgi?field=0&regexp=Journal+of+Speech,+Language,+and+Hearing+Research+:+Jslhr&dispmax=20&dispstart=0

- **Panminerva Medica. (Panminerva Med)**
  http://www.ncbi.nlm.nih.gov/entrez/jrbrowser.cgi?field=0&regexp=Panminerva+Medica&dispmax=20&dispstart=0

CHAPTER 8. PHYSICIAN GUIDELINES AND DATABASES

Overview

Doctors and medical researchers rely on a number of information sources to help patients with their conditions. Many will subscribe to journals or newsletters published by their professional associations or refer to specialized textbooks or clinical guides published for the medical profession. In this chapter, we focus on databases and Internet-based guidelines created or written for this professional audience.

NIH Guidelines

For the more common diseases, The National Institutes of Health publish guidelines that are frequently consulted by physicians. Publications are typically written by one or more of the various NIH Institutes. For physician guidelines, commonly referred to as "clinical" or "professional" guidelines, you can visit the following Institutes:

- Office of the Director (OD); guidelines consolidated across agencies available at **http://www.nih.gov/health/consumer/conkey.htm**

- National Institute of General Medical Sciences (NIGMS); fact sheets available at **http://www.nigms.nih.gov/news/facts/**

- National Library of Medicine (NLM); extensive encyclopedia (A.D.A.M., Inc.) with guidelines:
  http://www.nlm.nih.gov/medlineplus/healthtopics.html

- National Institute on Deafness and Other Communication Disorders (NIDCD); fact sheets and guidelines at
  http://www.nidcd.nih.gov/health/health.htm

NIH Databases

In addition to the various Institutes of Health that publish professional guidelines, the NIH has designed a number of databases for professionals.[25] Physician-oriented resources provide a wide variety of information related to the biomedical and health sciences, both past and present. The format of these resources varies. Searchable databases, bibliographic citations, full text articles (when available), archival collections, and images are all available. The following are referenced by the National Library of Medicine:[26]

- **Bioethics:** Access to published literature on the ethical, legal and public policy issues surrounding healthcare and biomedical research. This information is provided in conjunction with the Kennedy Institute of Ethics located at Georgetown University, Washington, D.C.: **http://www.nlm.nih.gov/databases/databases_bioethics.html**

- **HIV/AIDS Resources:** Describes various links and databases dedicated to HIV/AIDS research: **http://www.nlm.nih.gov/pubs/factsheets/aidsinfs.html**

- **NLM Online Exhibitions:** Describes "Exhibitions in the History of Medicine": **http://www.nlm.nih.gov/exhibition/exhibition.html**. Additional resources for historical scholarship in medicine: **http://www.nlm.nih.gov/hmd/hmd.html**

- **Biotechnology Information:** Access to public databases. The National Center for Biotechnology Information conducts research in computational biology, develops software tools for analyzing genome data, and disseminates biomedical information for the better understanding of molecular processes affecting human health and disease: **http://www.ncbi.nlm.nih.gov/**

- **Population Information:** The National Library of Medicine provides access to worldwide coverage of population, family planning, and related health issues, including family planning technology and programs, fertility, and population law and policy: **http://www.nlm.nih.gov/databases/databases_population.html**

- **Cancer Information:** Access to caner-oriented databases: **http://www.nlm.nih.gov/databases/databases_cancer.html**

---

[25] Remember, for the general public, the National Library of Medicine recommends the databases referenced in MEDLINE*plus* (**http://medlineplus.gov/** or **http://www.nlm.nih.gov/medlineplus/databases.html**).
[26] See **http://www.nlm.nih.gov/databases/databases.html**.

- **Profiles in Science:** Offering the archival collections of prominent twentieth-century biomedical scientists to the public through modern digital technology: **http://www.profiles.nlm.nih.gov/**

- **Chemical Information:** Provides links to various chemical databases and references: **http://sis.nlm.nih.gov/Chem/ChemMain.html**

- **Clinical Alerts:** Reports the release of findings from the NIH-funded clinical trials where such release could significantly affect morbidity and mortality: **http://www.nlm.nih.gov/databases/alerts/clinical_alerts.html**

- **Space Life Sciences:** Provides links and information to space-based research (including NASA): **http://www.nlm.nih.gov/databases/databases_space.html**

- **MEDLINE:** Bibliographic database covering the fields of medicine, nursing, dentistry, veterinary medicine, the healthcare system, and the pre-clinical sciences: **http://www.nlm.nih.gov/databases/databases_medline.html**

- **Toxicology and Environmental Health Information (TOXNET):** Databases covering toxicology and environmental health: **http://sis.nlm.nih.gov/Tox/ToxMain.html**

- **Visible Human Interface:** Anatomically detailed, three-dimensional representations of normal male and female human bodies: **http://www.nlm.nih.gov/research/visible/visible_human.html**

While all of the above references may be of interest to physicians who study and treat aphasia, the following are particularly noteworthy.

The Combined Health Information Database

A comprehensive source of information on clinical guidelines written for professionals is the Combined Health Information Database. You will need to limit your search to "Brochure/Pamphlet," "Fact Sheet," or "Information Package" and aphasia using the "Detailed Search" option. Go directly to the following hyperlink: **http://chid.nih.gov/detail/detail.html**. To find associations, use the drop boxes at the bottom of the search page where "You may refine your search by." For the publication date, select "All Years," select your preferred language, and the format option "Fact Sheet." By making these selections and typing "aphasia" (or synonyms) into the "For these words:" box above, you will only receive results on fact sheets dealing with aphasia. The following is a sample result:

- **Communication for a Lifetime: Speech, Language, and Hearing in the Older Adult**

Source: Rockville, MD: American Speech-Language-Hearing Association (ASHA). 200x. 12 p.

Contact: Available from American Speech-Language-Hearing Association (ASHA). Product Sales, 10801 Rockville Pike, Rockville, MD 20852. (888) 498-6699. TTY (301) 897-0157. Website: www.asha.org. PRICE: $4.00 for 10, plus shipping and handling. Item Number: 0210105.

Summary: This brochure reviews the typical changes in communication abilities that can accompany aging. The brochure emphasizes that knowing about speech, language, and hearing disorders can prevent or reduce the impact of any losses and enhance the ability to continue a happy and healthy life. The brochure offers facts about aging and hearing loss, including the statistics of hearing loss, its typical causes, and the impact of hearing loss on everyday life. The brochure then reviews the same type of information for speech and language disorders, including aphasia (reduced understanding of language), dysarthria (a nervous system of muscle disorder that makes speech hard for others to understand), apraxia of speech (difficulty coordinating the muscles of speech), cognitive communication impairments, laryngectomy (removal of the larynx, or voice box), and dysphagia (swallowing disorder). The brochure concludes by encouraging readers who have concerns about speech language or swallowing impairments to consult a speech language pathologist for an evaluation and appropriate recommendations. The brochure briefly summarizes the role of audiologists and speech language pathologists, and how to find an appropriate certified professional. The contact information for the American Speech Language Hearing Association (ASHA) is provided.

- **About Speech and Language Disorders**

Source: South Deerfield, MA: Channing L. Bete Company, Inc. 1997. 16 p.

Contact: Available from Channing L. Bete Company, Inc. 200 State Road, South Deerfield, MA 01373. (800) 628-7733 or (413) 665-7611; Fax (800) 499-6464; http://www.channing.bete.com. PRICE: $1.25 for 1-24 copies; bulk rates available. Item Number 12542F-3-96.

Summary: This health education booklet familiarizes readers with speech and language disorders. Defined as difficulties in understanding or expressing thoughts, the booklet explains speech and language disorders and how they can affect learning, independence, relationships, and emotional well-being. The booklet outlines the three aspects of normal communication: hearing, interpreting, and speaking. Communication disorders can result from physical problems, health problems, learning problems, and other problems such as mental retardation, low self-esteem, or emotional disturbances. Specific speech and language disorders outlined include stuttering, poor voice control, articulation disorders, aphasia, learning disabilities, dysarthria, and loss of voice. The early warning signs of speech and language disorders in children include slow development, speech problems, learning disabilities, and behavioral problems; the brochure emphasizes the importance of early identification. The brochure concludes with information about the role of the speech language pathologist, treatment options, where to get additional information about speech and language problems, and the important role of the school. The brochure is illustrated with simple cartoon drawings of families and children.

- **Dysarthria: Understanding This Speech Problem**

Source: San Bruno, CA: Krames Communications. 1997. [4 p.].

Contact: Available from Krames Communications. Order Department, 1100 Grundy Lane, San Bruno, CA 94066-9821. (800) 333-3032; Fax (415) 244-4512. PRICE: Single copy free; $20.00 per pack of 50 brochures. Item Number 9433-LNZL.

Summary: This brochure explains dysarthria, a speech problem caused by a lack of control over muscles in the face and mouth. This problem may occur when the brain is damaged by injury or illness. A person who has dysarthria knows which words to use, but may not be able to make the right sounds. The brochure lists the common signs of dysarthria and describes the role of speech language therapy in the rehabilitation work of persons with dysarthria. The brochure includes a sidebar offering strategies for family members or caregivers who wish to help the person with dysarthria practice his or her communication skills. The brochure is illustrated with full-color drawings of patients in speech therapy settings. One section briefly describes the related problems of aphasia (trouble using language) and dysphagia (swallowing difficulty).

- **Traumatic Brain Injury: A Guide for the Patient and Family**

Source: Stow, OH: Interactive Therapeutics, Inc. 1993. 61 p.

Contact: Available from Interactive Therapeutics, Inc. P.O. Box 1805, Stow, OH 44224. (800) 253-5111 or (216) 688-1371; Fax (330) 923-3030; E-mail: winteract@aol.com. PRICE: $4.50 each for 1 to 25 copies; bulk rates available.

Summary: This booklet is intended to serve as an introduction to traumatic brain injury (TBI) and as a reference to other sources of information to guide patients and their families as they learn about TBI. Four sections cover brain function, TBI and how it affects the brain, what to expect during recovery and rehabilitation, and living and coping with TBI. The chapter on possible impairments from TBI includes a section on speech and language disorders, covering aphasia, communication problems, dysarthria, and apraxia of speech. The booklet concludes with an extensive glossary of terms.

- **Understanding Stroke**

  Source: Chicago, IL: National Easter Seal Society. 1992. [2 p.].

  Contact: Available from National Easter Seal Society. 230 West Monroe Street, Suite 1800, Chicago, IL 60606. Voice (312) 726-6200; TTY (708) 726-4258; Fax (312) 726-1494. PRICE: $7.50 per 25 copies. Order Number A-235.

  Summary: This brochure provides an overview of stroke, brain damage resulting from a blockage of, or hemorrhage from, the blood vessels to the brain. Topics include immediate post-stroke symptoms and recovery, the importance of patience on the part of family members and caregivers, the emotional impact of stroke, the warning signs and symptoms of stroke, and risk factors for stroke. The brochure defines related terms, including aphasia, cerebral embolism, cerebral hemorrhage, cerebral thrombosis, cerebral vascular accident (CVA), and hemianopia. The brochure is produced by the National Easter Seal Society, an organization founded to help people with disabilities achieve maximum independence.

- **Careers in Speech-Language Pathology and Audiology**

  Source: Rockville, MD: American Speech-Language-Hearing Association (ASHA). 1991. [2 p.].

  Contact: Available from American Speech-Language-Hearing Association (ASHA). Product Sales, 10801 Rockville Pike, Rockville, MD 20852. (888) 498-6699. TTY (301) 897-0157. Website: www.asha.org. PRICE: $3.75 for 10 copies; bulk rates available. Item Number 0111544.

  Summary: This brochure provides information about the professions of speech-language pathology and audiology. Speech-language pathology and audiology are concerned with evaluation, treatment, and research in human communication and its disorders. Speech language pathologists treat disorders such as stuttering, delayed language development, aphasia, and voice and articulation problems. Audiologists specialize in prevention, identification, assessment, and rehabilitation of hearing disorders. This brochure discusses the job outlook for the future, requirements for certification and licensure, and financial assistance for higher education. The brochure concludes with information about related professional organizations, including the American Speech Language Hearing Association (ASHA), and the National Student Speech Language Hearing Association (NSSLHA). The brochure is illustrated with full-color photographs of hearing specialists at work. (AA-M).

- **Communication Disorders and Aging**

Source: Rockville, MD: American Speech-Language-Hearing Association (ASHA). 199x. [2 p.].

Contact: Available from American Speech-Language-Hearing Association (ASHA). Product Sales, 10801 Rockville Pike, Rockville, MD 20852. (888) 498-6699. TTY (301) 897-0157. Website: www.asha.org. PRICE: Single copy free; bulk orders available. Item Number 0210105.

Summary: This brochure summarizes the communication disorders that most frequently affect older people. The brochure notes that with the number of older adults growing rapidly and an increased numbers of survivors of illnesses and accidents that can result in speech, language, or hearing disorders, there will be more adults with communication problems. The brochure describes why communication disorders can be especially serious in older adults, then summarizes five different disorders: aphasia, hearing problems, dysarthria, voice problems, and other communication problems associated with brain diseases. The brochure describes the roles of the speech-language pathologist and the audiologist and the differences between them. A final section describes where readers can locate speech, language, and audiology services. The brochure is illustrated with full-color photographs.

- **Recognizing Communication Disorders**

Source: Rockville, MD: American Speech-Language-Hearing Association (ASHA). 199x. [2 p.].

Contact: Available from American Speech-Language-Hearing Association (ASHA). Product Sales, 10801 Rockville Pike, Rockville, MD 20852. (888) 498-6699. TTY (301) 897-0157. Website: www.asha.org. PRICE: Single copy free; bulk orders available. Item Number 0210104.

Summary: This brochure familiarizes readers with communication disorders, including hearing disorders and speech and language disorders. The brochure stresses that human communication is essential to learning, working, and social interaction; therefore, impaired communication can affect every aspect of a person's life. Topics include the signs of communication disorders; common hearing disorders, including conductive, sensorineural, and mixed hearing losses; common language disorders, including delayed language and aphasia; common speech disorders, including stuttering, articulation disorders, and voice disorders; the causes of communication disorders; the roles of the speech-language pathologist and the audiologist and the differences between them; and how to locate speech language and audiology services. The brochure concludes with a list of brochures available from ASHA.

- **Effective Communication with the Aphasic Person**

  Source: Englewood, CO: National Stroke Association. 199x. 8 p.

  Contact: National Stroke Association. 8480 East Orchard Road, Englewood, CO 80111-5015. (303) 771-1700. PRICE: Single copy free.

  Summary: This pamphlet describes aphasia, which is an impairment in language and communication ability due to brain injury. The publication educates caregivers and family about how to communicate with people who have aphasia. The pamphlet discusses the communication difficulties that individuals with aphasia have in listening and understanding language, gesturing, reading, and speaking. The document lists additional materials concerning stroke and recovering from a stroke.

- **Speech-Language Pathologists: Helping People Find the Words**

  Source: Rockville, MD: American Speech-Hearing-Language Association (ASHA). 199x. [2 p.].

  Contact: Available from American Speech-Language-Hearing Association (ASHA). Product Sales, 10801 Rockville Pike, Rockville, MD 20852. (888) 498-6699. TTY (301) 897-0157. Website: www.asha.org. PRICE: $10.00 for 50, plus shipping and handling. Item Number: 0111645.

  Summary: This brochure familiarizes readers with the services provided by speech language pathologists. The brochure defines certified speech language pathologists as the professionals who identify, evaluate, and treat a wide range of speech, language, and swallowing disorders. The brochure lists and briefly defines the disorders that might be dealt with by the speech language therapist: stuttering, articulation disorders, language disorders, aphasia, voice disorders, cognitive communication disorders, and swallowing disorders (dysphagia). The brochure then describes augmentative and alternative communication, and communication enhancement strategies. The brochure includes quotations from patients who have been helped by speech language therapy. The back cover of the brochure explains the certification and professional education requirements of the certified speech language pathologist. 2 figures.

- **Speech-Language Pathology: Helping Your Patients with Speech, Language or Swallowing Disorders**

  Source: Rockville, MD: American Speech-Language-Hearing Association (ASHA). 199x. [2 p.].

  Contact: Available from American Speech-Language-Hearing Association (ASHA). Action Center, 10801 Rockville Pike, Rockville, MD 20852. (800) 638-8255. E-mail: actioncenter@asha.org. Website: www.asha.org. PRICE: Single copy free for members.

  Summary: A speech language pathologist is the health care professional educated and trained to evaluate and treat children and adults with speech, language, and swallowing problems. This brochure, from the American Speech Language Hearing Association (ASHA), reviews the services that speech language pathologists provide, and reminds physicians and other health care providers of the situations where referral to a speech language pathologist can be helpful for their patients. The brochure reviews common types of speech language disorders, including articulation disorders, language disorders, aphasia (loss of the ability to comprehend words), stuttering, voice disorders, cognitive communication disorders, and dysphagia (swallowing difficulty), with a focus on the services that speech language pathologists can provide to patients with each type of disorder. Speech language pathologists are also trained to offer new possibilities for people with communication disorders through augmentative and alternative communication, including voice synthesizing computers and communication boards. The brochure concludes with the contact information for ASHA and a description of the certification process for speech language pathologists. The brochure is illustrated with black and white photographs of speech language pathologists at work. 3 figures.

The NLM Gateway[27]

The NLM (National Library of Medicine) Gateway is a Web-based system that lets users search simultaneously in multiple retrieval systems at the U.S. National Library of Medicine (NLM). It allows users of NLM services to initiate searches from one Web interface, providing "one-stop searching" for

---

[27] Adapted from NLM: **http://gateway.nlm.nih.gov/gw/Cmd?Overview.x**.

many of NLM's information resources or databases.[28] One target audience for the Gateway is the Internet user who is new to NLM's online resources and does not know what information is available or how best to search for it. This audience may include physicians and other healthcare providers, researchers, librarians, students, and, increasingly, patients, their families, and the public.[29] To use the NLM Gateway, simply go to the search site at **http://gateway.nlm.nih.gov/gw/Cmd**. Type "aphasia" (or synonyms) into the search box and click "Search." The results will be presented in a tabular form, indicating the number of references in each database category.

Results Summary

Category	Items Found
Journal Articles	8066
Books / Periodicals / Audio Visual	546
Consumer Health	50
Meeting Abstracts	12
Other Collections	1
Total	8675

HSTAT[30]

HSTAT is a free, Web-based resource that provides access to full-text documents used in healthcare decision-making.[31] HSTAT's audience includes healthcare providers, health service researchers, policy makers, insurance companies, consumers, and the information professionals who serve these groups. HSTAT provides access to a wide variety of publications, including clinical practice guidelines, quick-reference guides for clinicians,

---

[28] The NLM Gateway is currently being developed by the Lister Hill National Center for Biomedical Communications (LHNCBC) at the National Library of Medicine (NLM) of the National Institutes of Health (NIH).

[29] Other users may find the Gateway useful for an overall search of NLM's information resources. Some searchers may locate what they need immediately, while others will utilize the Gateway as an adjunct tool to other NLM search services such as PubMed® and MEDLINEplus®. The Gateway connects users with multiple NLM retrieval systems while also providing a search interface for its own collections. These collections include various types of information that do not logically belong in PubMed, LOCATORplus, or other established NLM retrieval systems (e.g., meeting announcements and pre-1966 journal citations). The Gateway will provide access to the information found in an increasing number of NLM retrieval systems in several phases.

[30] Adapted from HSTAT: **http://www.nlm.nih.gov/pubs/factsheets/hstat.html**

[31] The HSTAT URL is **http://hstat.nlm.nih.gov/**.

consumer health brochures, evidence reports and technology assessments from the Agency for Healthcare Research and Quality (AHRQ), as well as AHRQ's Put Prevention Into Practice.[32] Simply search by "aphasia" (or synonyms) at the following Web site: **http://text.nlm.nih.gov**.

Coffee Break: Tutorials for Biologists[33]

Some patients may wish to have access to a general healthcare site that takes a scientific view of the news and covers recent breakthroughs in biology that may one day assist physicians in developing treatments. To this end, we recommend "Coffee Break," a collection of short reports on recent biological discoveries. Each report incorporates interactive tutorials that demonstrate how bioinformatics tools are used as a part of the research process. Currently, all Coffee Breaks are written by NCBI staff.[34] Each report is about 400 words and is usually based on a discovery reported in one or more articles from recently published, peer-reviewed literature.[35] This site has new articles every few weeks, so it can be considered an online magazine of sorts, and intended for general background information. You can access the Coffee Break Web site at **http://www.ncbi.nlm.nih.gov/Coffeebreak/**.

---

[32] Other important documents in HSTAT include: the National Institutes of Health (NIH) Consensus Conference Reports and Technology Assessment Reports; the HIV/AIDS Treatment Information Service (ATIS) resource documents; the Substance Abuse and Mental Health Services Administration's Center for Substance Abuse Treatment (SAMHSA/CSAT) Treatment Improvement Protocols (TIP) and Center for Substance Abuse Prevention (SAMHSA/CSAP) Prevention Enhancement Protocols System (PEPS); the Public Health Service (PHS) Preventive Services Task Force's *Guide to Clinical Preventive Services*; the independent, nonfederal Task Force on Community Services *Guide to Community Preventive Services*; and the Health Technology Advisory Committee (HTAC) of the Minnesota Health Care Commission (MHCC) health technology evaluations.

[33] Adapted from **http://www.ncbi.nlm.nih.gov/Coffeebreak/Archive/FAQ.html**

[34] The figure that accompanies each article is frequently supplied by an expert external to NCBI, in which case the source of the figure is cited. The result is an interactive tutorial that tells a biological story.

[35] After a brief introduction that sets the work described into a broader context, the report focuses on how a molecular understanding can provide explanations of observed biology and lead to therapies for diseases. Each vignette is accompanied by a figure and hypertext links that lead to a series of pages that interactively show how NCBI tools and resources are used in the research process.

Other Commercial Databases

In addition to resources maintained by official agencies, other databases exist that are commercial ventures addressing medical professionals. Here are a few examples that may interest you:

- **CliniWeb International:** Index and table of contents to selected clinical information on the Internet; see **http://www.ohsu.edu/cliniweb/**.

- **Image Engine:** Multimedia electronic medical record system that integrates a wide range of digitized clinical images with textual data stored in the University of Pittsburgh Medical Center's MARS electronic medical record system; see the following Web site: **http://www.cml.upmc.edu/cml/imageengine/imageEngine.html**.

- **Medical World Search:** Searches full text from thousands of selected medical sites on the Internet; see **http://www.mwsearch.com/**.

- **MedWeaver:** Prototype system that allows users to search differential diagnoses for any list of signs and symptoms, to search medical literature, and to explore relevant Web sites; see **http://www.med.virginia.edu/~wmd4n/medweaver.html**.

- **Metaphrase:** Middleware component intended for use by both caregivers and medical records personnel. It converts the informal language generally used by caregivers into terms from formal, controlled vocabularies; see **http://www.lexical.com/Metaphrase.html**.

The Genome Project and Aphasia

With all the discussion in the press about the Human Genome Project, it is only natural that physicians, researchers, and patients want to know about how human genes relate to aphasia. In the following section, we will discuss databases and references used by physicians and scientists who work in this area.

Online Mendelian Inheritance in Man (OMIM)

The Online Mendelian Inheritance in Man (OMIM) database is a catalog of human genes and genetic disorders authored and edited by Dr. Victor A. McKusick and his colleagues at Johns Hopkins and elsewhere. OMIM was developed for the World Wide Web by the National Center for

Biotechnology Information (NCBI).[36] The database contains textual information, pictures, and reference information. It also contains copious links to NCBI's Entrez database of MEDLINE articles and sequence information.

Go to **http://www.ncbi.nlm.nih.gov/Omim/searchomim.html** To search the database. Type "aphasia" (or synonyms) in the search box, and click "Submit Search." If too many results appear, you can narrow the search by adding the word "clinical." Each report will have additional links to related research and databases. By following these links, especially the link titled "Database Links," you will be exposed to numerous specialized databases that are largely used by the scientific community. These databases are overly technical and seldom used by the general public, but offer an abundance of information. The following is an example of the results you can obtain from the OMIM for aphasia:

- **Mental Retardation, X-linked Nonspecific, with Aphasia**
  Web site: http://www.ncbi.nlm.nih.gov/htbin-post/Omim/dispmim?309545

Genes and Disease (NCBI - Map)

The Genes and Disease database is produced by the National Center for Biotechnology Information of the National Library of Medicine at the National Institutes of Health. Go to **http://www.ncbi.nlm.nih.gov/disease/**, and browse the system pages to have a full view of important conditions linked to human genes. Since this site is regularly updated, you may wish to re-visit it from time to time. The following systems and associated disorders are addressed:

- **Immune System:** Fights invaders.
  Examples: Asthma, autoimmune polyglandular syndrome, Crohn's disease, DiGeorge syndrome, familial Mediterranean fever, immunodeficiency with Hyper-IgM, severe combined immunodeficiency.
  Web site: **http://www.ncbi.nlm.nih.gov/disease/Immune.html**

- **Muscle and Bone:** Movement and growth.
  Examples: Duchenne muscular dystrophy, Ellis-van Creveld syndrome,

---

[36] Adapted from **http://www.ncbi.nlm.nih.gov/**. Established in 1988 as a national resource for molecular biology information, NCBI creates public databases, conducts research in computational biology, develops software tools for analyzing genome data, and disseminates biomedical information--all for the better understanding of molecular processes affecting human health and disease.

Marfan syndrome, myotonic dystrophy, spinal muscular atrophy.
Web site: **http://www.ncbi.nlm.nih.gov/disease/Muscle.html**

- **Nervous System:** Mind and body.
Examples: Alzheimer disease, Amyotrophic lateral sclerosis, Angelman syndrome, Charcot-Marie-Tooth disease, epilepsy, essential tremor, Fragile X syndrome, Friedreich's ataxia, Huntington disease, Niemann-Pick disease, Parkinson disease, Prader-Willi syndrome, Rett syndrome, Spinocerebellar atrophy, Williams syndrome.
Web site: **http://www.ncbi.nlm.nih.gov/disease/Brain.html**

- **Signals:** Cellular messages.
Examples: Ataxia telangiectasia, Baldness, Cockayne syndrome, Glaucoma, SRY: sex determination, Tuberous sclerosis, Waardenburg syndrome, Werner syndrome.
Web site: **http://www.ncbi.nlm.nih.gov/disease/Signals.html**

- **Transporters:** Pumps and channels.
Examples: Cystic Fibrosis, deafness, diastrophic dysplasia, Hemophilia A, long-QT syndrome, Menkes syndrome, Pendred syndrome, polycystic kidney disease, sickle cell anemia, Wilson's disease, Zellweger syndrome.
Web site: **http://www.ncbi.nlm.nih.gov/disease/Transporters.html**

Entrez

Entrez is a search and retrieval system that integrates several linked databases at the National Center for Biotechnology Information (NCBI). These databases include nucleotide sequences, protein sequences, macromolecular structures, whole genomes, and MEDLINE through PubMed. Entrez provides access to the following databases:

- **PubMed:** Biomedical literature (PubMed),
Web site: **http://www.ncbi.nlm.nih.gov/entrez/query.fcgi?db=PubMed**

- **Nucleotide Sequence Database (Genbank):**
Web site:
http://www.ncbi.nlm.nih.gov/entrez/query.fcgi?db=Nucleotide

- **Protein Sequence Database:**
Web site: **http://www.ncbi.nlm.nih.gov/entrez/query.fcgi?db=Protein**

- **Structure:** Three-dimensional macromolecular structures,
Web site: **http://www.ncbi.nlm.nih.gov/entrez/query.fcgi?db=Structure**

- **Genome:** Complete genome assemblies,
Web site: **http://www.ncbi.nlm.nih.gov/entrez/query.fcgi?db=Genome**

- **PopSet:** Population study data sets,
  Web site: **http://www.ncbi.nlm.nih.gov/entrez/query.fcgi?db=Popset**

- **OMIM:** Online Mendelian Inheritance in Man,
  Web site: **http://www.ncbi.nlm.nih.gov/entrez/query.fcgi?db=OMIM**

- **Taxonomy:** Organisms in GenBank,
  Web site:
  http://www.ncbi.nlm.nih.gov/entrez/query.fcgi?db=Taxonomy

- **Books:** Online books,
  Web site: **http://www.ncbi.nlm.nih.gov/entrez/query.fcgi?db=books**

- **ProbeSet:** Gene Expression Omnibus (GEO),
  Web site: **http://www.ncbi.nlm.nih.gov/entrez/query.fcgi?db=geo**

- **3D Domains:** Domains from Entrez Structure,
  Web site: **http://www.ncbi.nlm.nih.gov/entrez/query.fcgi?db=geo**

- **NCBI's Protein Sequence Information Survey Results:**
  Web site: **http://www.ncbi.nlm.nih.gov/About/proteinsurvey/**

To access the Entrez system at the National Center for Biotechnology Information, go to **http://www.ncbi.nlm.nih.gov/entrez**, and then select the database that you would like to search. The databases available are listed in the drop box next to "Search." In the box next to "for," enter "aphasia" (or synonyms) and click "Go."

Jablonski's Multiple Congenital Anomaly/Mental Retardation (MCA/MR) Syndromes Database[37]

This online resource can be quite useful. It has been developed to facilitate the identification and differentiation of syndromic entities. Special attention is given to the type of information that is usually limited or completely omitted in existing reference sources due to space limitations of the printed form.

At **http://www.nlm.nih.gov/mesh/jablonski/syndrome_toc/toc_a.html** you can also search across syndromes using an alphabetical index. You can also search at **http://www.nlm.nih.gov/mesh/jablonski/syndrome_db.html**.

---

[37] Adapted from the National Library of Medicine:
http://www.nlm.nih.gov/mesh/jablonski/about_syndrome.html.

The Genome Database[38]

Established at Johns Hopkins University in Baltimore, Maryland in 1990, the Genome Database (GDB) is the official central repository for genomic mapping data resulting from the Human Genome Initiative. In the spring of 1999, the Bioinformatics Supercomputing Centre (BiSC) at the Hospital for Sick Children in Toronto, Ontario assumed the management of GDB. The Human Genome Initiative is a worldwide research effort focusing on structural analysis of human DNA to determine the location and sequence of the estimated 100,000 human genes. In support of this project, GDB stores and curates data generated by researchers worldwide who are engaged in the mapping effort of the Human Genome Project (HGP). GDB's mission is to provide scientists with an encyclopedia of the human genome which is continually revised and updated to reflect the current state of scientific knowledge. Although GDB has historically focused on gene mapping, its focus will broaden as the Genome Project moves from mapping to sequence, and finally, to functional analysis.

To access the GDB, simply go to the following hyperlink: **http://www.gdb.org/**. Search "All Biological Data" by "Keyword." Type "aphasia" (or synonyms) into the search box, and review the results. If more than one word is used in the search box, then separate each one with the word "and" or "or" (using "or" might be useful when using synonyms). This database is extremely technical as it was created for specialists. The articles are the results which are the most accessible to non-professionals and often listed under the heading "Citations." The contact names are also accessible to non-professionals.

Specialized References

The following books are specialized references written for professionals interested in aphasia (sorted alphabetically by title, hyperlinks provide rankings, information, and reviews at Amazon.com):

- **Assessment in Speech-Language Pathology: A Resource Manual** by Kenneth G. Shipley, Julie G. McAfee; Spiral-bound - 424 pages, 2nd edition (March 1, 1998), Singular Publishing Group; ISBN: 1565938704; **http://www.amazon.com/exec/obidos/ASIN/1565938704/icongroupinterna**

- **Augmentative and Alternative Communication for Adults with Acquired Neurologic Disorders** by David R. Beukelman, Ph.D. (Editor), et

---

[38] Adapted from the Genome Database:
http://gdbwww.gdb.org/gdb/aboutGDB.html#mission.

al; Hardcover – 448 pages (July 2000), Paul H Brookes Publishing Co.; ISBN: 1557664730; http://www.amazon.com/exec/obidos/ASIN/1557664730/icongroupinterna

- **Central Auditory Processing Disorders: Mostly Management** by M. Gay Masters, et al; Hardcover - 288 pages, 1st edition (April 7, 1998), Allyn & Bacon; ISBN: 0205273610; http://www.amazon.com/exec/obidos/ASIN/0205273610/icongroupinterna

- **Cognitive-Communication Disorders Following Traumatic Brain Injury : A Practical Guide** by Jane Freund, et al; Paperback – 138 pages (January 1999); Reissue edition, Psychological Corp; ISBN: 0127845844; http://www.amazon.com/exec/obidos/ASIN/0127845844/icongroupinterna

- **Counseling Individuals with Communication Disorders, Psychodynamic and Family Aspects** by Walter J. Rollin; Hardcover - 272 pages; 2nd edition (May 1, 2000), Butterworth-Heinemann Medical; ISBN: 0750671785; http://www.amazon.com/exec/obidos/ASIN/0750671785/icongroupinterna

- **Motor Speech Disorders** by Frederic L. Darley, et al; Hardcover (October 1997), W B Saunders Co.; ISBN: 0721628788; http://www.amazon.com/exec/obidos/ASIN/0721628788/icongroupinterna

- **Therapy Techniques for Cleft Palate Speech and Related Disorders** by Karen J. Golding-Kushner; Paperback - 175 pages; 1st edition, Singular Publishing Group; ISBN: 076930169X; http://www.amazon.com/exec/obidos/ASIN/076930169X/icongroupinterna

Vocabulary Builder

Audiology: The study of hearing and hearing impairment. [NIH]

Confusion: Disturbed orientation in regard to time, place, or person, sometimes accompanied by disordered consciousness. [EU]

Laryngectomy: Total or partial excision of the larynx. [NIH]

Larynx: An irregularly shaped, musculocartilaginous tubular structure, lined with mucous membrane, located at the top of the trachea and below the root of the tongue and the hyoid bone. It is the essential sphincter guarding the entrance into the trachea and functioning secondarily as the organ of voice. [NIH]

Molecular: Of, pertaining to, or composed of molecules : a very small mass of matter. [EU]

Mutism: Inability or refusal to speak. [EU]

Ototoxic: Having a deleterious effect upon the eighth nerve, or upon the organs of hearing and balance. [EU]

Phobia: A persistent, irrational, intense fear of a specific object, activity, or situation (the phobic stimulus), fear that is recognized as being excessive or unreasonable by the individual himself. When a phobia is a significant source of distress or interferes with social functioning, it is considered a mental disorder; phobic disorder (or neurosis). In DSM III phobic disorders are subclassified as agoraphobia, social phobias, and simple phobias. Used as a word termination denoting irrational fear of or aversion to the subject indicated by the stem to which it is affixed. [EU]

Prejudice: A preconceived judgment made without adequate evidence and not easily alterable by presentation of contrary evidence. [NIH]

Vertigo: An illusion of movement; a sensation as if the external world were revolving around the patient (objective vertigo) or as if he himself were revolving in space (subjective vertigo). The term is sometimes erroneously used to mean any form of dizziness. [EU]

CHAPTER 9. DISSERTATIONS ON APHASIA

Overview

University researchers are active in studying almost all known diseases. The result of research is often published in the form of Doctoral or Master's dissertations. You should understand, therefore, that applied diagnostic procedures and/or therapies can take many years to develop after the thesis that proposed the new technique or approach was written.

In this chapter, we will give you a bibliography on recent dissertations relating to aphasia. You can read about these in more detail using the Internet or your local medical library. We will also provide you with information on how to use the Internet to stay current on dissertations.

Dissertations on Aphasia

ProQuest Digital Dissertations is the largest archive of academic dissertations available. From this archive, we have compiled the following list covering dissertations devoted to aphasia. You will see that the information provided includes the dissertation's title, its author, and the author's institution. To read more about the following, simply use the Internet address indicated. The following covers recent dissertations dealing with aphasia:

- **A Comparative Study of the Overall Validity of Tests Used for the Assessment of Bilingual/polyglot Aphasia with Particular Emphasis in German-english** by Migliozzi-kulik, Ria-margret, Edd from University of San Francisco, 1988, 356 pages
  http://wwwlib.umi.com/dissertations/fullcit/8900603

- **A Comparison of Spoken Language Abilities in Children with Aphasia, Autism, Learning Disabilities, and Normal Language Abilities** by Mcdonough, Dayle Davis, Phd from University of New Orleans, 1986, 162 pages
  http://wwwlib.umi.com/dissertations/fullcit/8625151

- **A Comparison of the Performance of Participants with and without Aphasia on an Environmental Symbol Recognition Task** by Davis, Janika Bullock; Ms from University of South Alabama, 2000, 58 pages
  http://wwwlib.umi.com/dissertations/fullcit/1398256

- **A Cross-linguistic Study of Verb Inflections in Agrammatism (icelandic, Hindi, Finnish, Morphology, Aphasia)** by Lorch, Marjorie Perlman, Phd from Boston University, 1986, 136 pages
  http://wwwlib.umi.com/dissertations/fullcit/8602739

- **A Method of Assessing Nonverbal Communication in Global Aphasia** by Glickstein, Joan Katz, Phd from University of Pittsburgh, 1979, 176 pages
  http://wwwlib.umi.com/dissertations/fullcit/8004859

- **A Neurolinguistic Description of Neologistic Jargon Aphasia.** by Buckingham, Hugh Woodstock, Jr., Phd from The University of Rochester, 1974, 235 pages
  http://wwwlib.umi.com/dissertations/fullcit/7515195

- **A Psycholinguistic Appraisal of Nonfluent Aphasia: a Case Study** by Dunlap, Anne Austin, Phd from State University of New York at Buffalo, 1981, 213 pages
  http://wwwlib.umi.com/dissertations/fullcit/8114667

- **A Semantic Analysis of Spontaneous Speech in Anomic Aphasia.** by Gordon, Karen Anne, Phd from State University of New York at Buffalo, 1975, 599 pages
  http://wwwlib.umi.com/dissertations/fullcit/7601440

- **A Study of Attention Allocation in Individuals with Aphasia** by Green, Carrie Cathleen; Ms from Texas Woman's University, 2000, 71 pages
  http://wwwlib.umi.com/dissertations/fullcit/1400307

- **Amnesic Aphasia and Goldstein's Holistic Method: an Epistemological Study.** by Di Piazza, Joseph Salvatore, Phd from University of Toronto (canada), 1973
  http://wwwlib.umi.com/dissertations/fullcit/f4543382

Keeping Current

As previously mentioned, an effective way to stay current on dissertations dedicated to aphasia is to use the database called *ProQuest Digital Dissertations* via the Internet, located at the following Web address: **http://wwwlib.umi.com/dissertations.** The site allows you to freely access the last two years of citations and abstracts. Ask your medical librarian if the library has full and unlimited access to this database. From the library, you should be able to do more complete searches than with the limited 2-year access available to the general public.

PART III. APPENDICES

ABOUT PART III

Part III is a collection of appendices on general medical topics which may be of interest to patients with aphasia and related conditions.

APPENDIX A. RESEARCHING YOUR MEDICATIONS

Overview

There are a number of sources available on new or existing medications which could be prescribed to patients with aphasia. While a number of hard copy or CD-Rom resources are available to patients and physicians for research purposes, a more flexible method is to use Internet-based databases. In this chapter, we will begin with a general overview of medications. We will then proceed to outline official recommendations on how you should view your medications. You may also want to research medications that you are currently taking for other conditions as they may interact with medications for aphasia. Research can give you information on the side effects, interactions, and limitations of prescription drugs used in the treatment of aphasia. Broadly speaking, there are two sources of information on approved medications: public sources and private sources. We will emphasize free-to-use public sources.

Your Medications: The Basics[39]

The Agency for Health Care Research and Quality has published extremely useful guidelines on how you can best participate in the medication aspects of aphasia. Taking medicines is not always as simple as swallowing a pill. It can involve many steps and decisions each day. The AHCRQ recommends that patients with aphasia take part in treatment decisions. Do not be afraid to ask questions and talk about your concerns. By taking a moment to ask questions early, you may avoid problems later. Here are some points to cover each time a new medicine is prescribed:

- Ask about all parts of your treatment, including diet changes, exercise, and medicines.

- Ask about the risks and benefits of each medicine or other treatment you might receive.

- Ask how often you or your doctor will check for side effects from a given medication.

Do not hesitate to ask what is important to you about your medicines. You may want a medicine with the fewest side effects, or the fewest doses to take each day. You may care most about cost, or how the medicine might affect how you live or work. Or, you may want the medicine your doctor believes will work the best. Telling your doctor will help him or her select the best treatment for you.

Do not be afraid to "bother" your doctor with your concerns and questions about medications for aphasia. You can also talk to a nurse or a pharmacist. They can help you better understand your treatment plan. Feel free to bring a friend or family member with you when you visit your doctor. Talking over your options with someone you trust can help you make better choices, especially if you are not feeling well. Specifically, ask your doctor the following:

- The name of the medicine and what it is supposed to do.

- How and when to take the medicine, how much to take, and for how long.

- What food, drinks, other medicines, or activities you should avoid while taking the medicine.

- What side effects the medicine may have, and what to do if they occur.

- If you can get a refill, and how often.

---

[39] This section is adapted from AHCRQ: **http://www.ahcpr.gov/consumer/ncpiebro.htm** .

- About any terms or directions you do not understand.

- What to do if you miss a dose.

- If there is written information you can take home (most pharmacies have information sheets on your prescription medicines; some even offer large-print or Spanish versions).

Do not forget to tell your doctor about all the medicines you are currently taking (not just those for aphasia). This includes prescription medicines and the medicines that you buy over the counter. Then your doctor can avoid giving you a new medicine that may not work well with the medications you take now. When talking to your doctor, you may wish to prepare a list of medicines you currently take, the reason you take them, and how you take them. Be sure to include the following information for each:

- Name of medicine

- Reason taken

- Dosage

- Time(s) of day

Also include any over-the-counter medicines, such as:

- Laxatives

- Diet pills

- Vitamins

- Cold medicine

- Aspirin or other pain, headache, or fever medicine

- Cough medicine

- Allergy relief medicine

- Antacids

- Sleeping pills

- Others (include names)

Learning More about Your Medications

Because of historical investments by various organizations and the emergence of the Internet, it has become rather simple to learn about the medications your doctor has recommended for aphasia. One such source is the United States Pharmacopeia. In 1820, eleven physicians met in Washington, D.C. to establish the first compendium of standard drugs for the United States. They called this compendium the "U.S. Pharmacopeia (USP)." Today, the USP is a non-profit organization consisting of 800 volunteer scientists, eleven elected officials, and 400 representatives of state associations and colleges of medicine and pharmacy. The USP is located in Rockville, Maryland, and its home page is located at **www.usp.org**. The USP currently provides standards for over 3,700 medications. The resulting USP DI® Advice for the Patient® can be accessed through the National Library of Medicine of the National Institutes of Health. The database is partially derived from lists of federally approved medications in the Food and Drug Administration's (FDA) Drug Approvals database.[40]

While the FDA database is rather large and difficult to navigate, the Phamacopeia is both user-friendly and free to use. It covers more than 9,000 prescription and over-the-counter medications. To access this database, simply type the following hyperlink into your Web browser: **http://www.nlm.nih.gov/medlineplus/druginformation.html**. To view examples of a given medication (brand names, category, description, preparation, proper use, precautions, side effects, etc.), simply follow the hyperlinks indicated within the United States Pharmacopoeia (USP). It is important to read the disclaimer by the USP (**http://www.nlm.nih.gov/medlineplus/drugdisclaimer.html**) before using the information provided.

Commercial Databases

In addition to the medications listed in the USP above, a number of commercial sites are available by subscription to physicians and their institutions. You may be able to access these sources from your local medical library or your doctor's office.

Reuters Health Drug Database

The Reuters Health Drug Database can be searched by keyword at the hyperlink: **http://www.reutershealth.com/frame2/drug.html**. The following medications are listed in the Reuters' database as associated with aphasia (including those with contraindications):[41]

---

[40] Though cumbersome, the FDA database can be freely browsed at the following site: **www.fda.gov/cder/da/da.htm**.

[41] Adapted from *A to Z Drug Facts* by Facts and Comparisons.

- **Donepezil**
  http://www.reutershealth.com/atoz/html/Donepezil.htm

- **Foscarnet Sodium**
  http://www.reutershealth.com/atoz/html/Foscarnet_Sodium.htm

- **Foscarnet Sodium (Phosphonoformic Acid)**
  http://www.reutershealth.com/atoz/html/Foscarnet_Sodium_(Phosphonoformic_Acid).htm

- **Methotrexate**
  http://www.reutershealth.com/atoz/html/Methotrexate.htm

- **Muromonab–CD3**
  http://www.reutershealth.com/atoz/html/Muromonab–CD3.htm

- **Rifabutin**
  http://www.reutershealth.com/atoz/html/Rifabutin.htm

- **Trazodone HCl**
  http://www.reutershealth.com/atoz/html/Trazodone_HCl.htm

Mosby's GenRx

Mosby's GenRx database (also available on CD-Rom and book format) covers 45,000 drug products including generics and international brands. It provides prescribing information, drug interactions, and patient information. Information in Mosby's GenRx database can be obtained at the following hyperlink: **http://www.genrx.com/Mosby/PhyGenRx/group.html**.

Physicians Desk Reference

The Physicians Desk Reference database (also available in CD-Rom and book format) is a full-text drug database. The database is searchable by brand name, generic name or by indication. It features multiple drug interactions reports. Information can be obtained at the following hyperlink: **http://physician.pdr.net/physician/templates/en/acl/psuser_t.htm**.

Other Web Sites

A number of additional Web sites discuss drug information. As an example, you may like to look at **www.drugs.com** which reproduces the information in the Pharmacopeia as well as commercial information. You may also want to consider the Web site of the Medical Letter, Inc. which allows users to download articles on various drugs and therapeutics for a nominal fee: **http://www.medletter.com/**.

Contraindications and Interactions (Hidden Dangers)

Some of the medications mentioned in the previous discussions can be problematic for patients with aphasia--not because they are used in the treatment process, but because of contraindications, or side effects. Medications with contraindications are those that could react with drugs used to treat aphasia or potentially create deleterious side effects in patients with aphasia. You should ask your physician about any contraindications, especially as these might apply to other medications that you may be taking for common ailments.

Drug-drug interactions occur when two or more drugs react with each other. This drug-drug interaction may cause you to experience an unexpected side effect. Drug interactions may make your medications less effective, cause unexpected side effects, or increase the action of a particular drug. Some drug interactions can even be harmful to you.

Be sure to read the label every time you use a nonprescription or prescription drug, and take the time to learn about drug interactions. These precautions may be critical to your health. You can reduce the risk of potentially harmful drug interactions and side effects with a little bit of knowledge and common sense.

Drug labels contain important information about ingredients, uses, warnings, and directions which you should take the time to read and understand. Labels also include warnings about possible drug interactions. Further, drug labels may change as new information becomes available. This is why it's especially important to read the label every time you use a medication. When your doctor prescribes a new drug, discuss all over-the-counter and prescription medications, dietary supplements, vitamins, botanicals, minerals and herbals you take as well as the foods you eat. Ask your pharmacist for the package insert for each prescription drug you take. The package insert provides more information about potential drug interactions.

A Final Warning

At some point, you may hear of alternative medications from friends, relatives, or in the news media. Advertisements may suggest that certain alternative drugs can produce positive results for patients with aphasia. Exercise caution--some of these drugs may have fraudulent claims, and others may actually hurt you. The Food and Drug Administration (FDA) is the official U.S. agency charged with discovering which medications are likely to improve the health of patients with aphasia. The FDA warns patients to watch out for[42]:

- Secret formulas (real scientists share what they know)

- Amazing breakthroughs or miracle cures (real breakthroughs don't happen very often; when they do, real scientists do not call them amazing or miracles)

- Quick, painless, or guaranteed cures

- If it sounds too good to be true, it probably isn't true.

If you have any questions about any kind of medical treatment, the FDA may have an office near you. Look for their number in the blue pages of the phone book. You can also contact the FDA through its toll-free number, 1-888-INFO-FDA (1-888-463-6332), or on the World Wide Web at **www.fda.gov**.

General References

In addition to the resources provided earlier in this chapter, the following general references describe medications (sorted alphabetically by title; hyperlinks provide rankings, information and reviews at Amazon.com):

- **Complete Guide to Prescription and Nonprescription Drugs 2001 (Complete Guide to Prescription and Nonprescription Drugs, 2001)** by H. Winter Griffith, Paperback 16th edition (2001), Medical Surveillance; ISBN: 0942447417;
  http://www.amazon.com/exec/obidos/ASIN/039952634X/icongroupinterna

- **The Effects of Drugs on Communication Disorders (Clinical Competence Series)** by Deanie Vogel, et al; Paperback - 248 pages; 2nd spiral edition (July 1999), Singular Publishing Group; ISBN: 1565939964;
  http://www.amazon.com/exec/obidos/ASIN/1565939964/icongroupinterna

---

[42] This section has been adapted from **http://www.fda.gov/opacom/lowlit/medfraud.html**

- **The Essential Guide to Prescription Drugs, 2001** by James J. Rybacki, James W. Long; Paperback - 1274 pages (2001), Harper Resource; ISBN: 0060958162;
  http://www.amazon.com/exec/obidos/ASIN/0060958162/icongroupinterna

- **Handbook of Commonly Prescribed Drugs** by G. John Digregorio, Edward J. Barbieri; Paperback 16th edition (2001), Medical Surveillance; ISBN: 0942447417;
  http://www.amazon.com/exec/obidos/ASIN/0942447417/icongroupinterna

- **Johns Hopkins Complete Home Encyclopedia of Drugs 2nd ed.** by Simeon Margolis (Ed.), Johns Hopkins; Hardcover - 835 pages (2000), Rebus; ISBN: 0929661583;
  http://www.amazon.com/exec/obidos/ASIN/0929661583/icongroupinterna

- **Medical Pocket Reference: Drugs 2002** by Springhouse Paperback 1st edition (2001), Lippincott Williams & Wilkins Publishers; ISBN: 1582550964;
  http://www.amazon.com/exec/obidos/ASIN/1582550964/icongroupinterna

- **PDR** by Medical Economics Staff, Medical Economics Staff Hardcover - 3506 pages 55th edition (2000), Medical Economics Company; ISBN: 1563633752;
  http://www.amazon.com/exec/obidos/ASIN/1563633752/icongroupinterna

- **Pharmacy Simplified: A Glossary of Terms** by James Grogan; Paperback - 432 pages, 1st edition (2001), Delmar Publishers; ISBN: 0766828581;
  http://www.amazon.com/exec/obidos/ASIN/0766828581/icongroupinterna

- **Physician Federal Desk Reference** by Christine B. Fraizer; Paperback 2nd edition (2001), Medicode Inc; ISBN: 1563373971;
  http://www.amazon.com/exec/obidos/ASIN/1563373971/icongroupinterna

- **Physician's Desk Reference Supplements** Paperback - 300 pages, 53 edition (1999), ISBN: 1563632950;
  http://www.amazon.com/exec/obidos/ASIN/1563632950/icongroupinterna

Vocabulary Builder

The following vocabulary builder gives definitions of words used in this chapter that have not been defined in previous chapters:

Methotrexate: An antineoplastic antimetabolite with immunosuppressant properties. It is an inhibitor of dihydrofolate reductase and prevents the formation of tetrahydrofolate, necessary for synthesis of thymidylate, an essential component of DNA. [NIH]

APPENDIX B. RESEARCHING ALTERNATIVE MEDICINE

Overview

Complementary and alternative medicine (CAM) is one of the most contentious aspects of modern medical practice. You may have heard of these treatments on the radio or on television. Maybe you have seen articles written about these treatments in magazines, newspapers, or books. Perhaps your friends or doctor have mentioned alternatives.

In this chapter, we will begin by giving you a broad perspective on complementary and alternative therapies. Next, we will introduce you to official information sources on CAM relating to aphasia. Finally, at the conclusion of this chapter, we will provide a list of readings on aphasia from various authors. We will begin, however, with the National Center for Complementary and Alternative Medicine's (NCCAM) overview of complementary and alternative medicine.

What Is CAM?[43]

Complementary and alternative medicine (CAM) covers a broad range of healing philosophies, approaches, and therapies. Generally, it is defined as those treatments and healthcare practices which are not taught in medical schools, used in hospitals, or reimbursed by medical insurance companies. Many CAM therapies are termed "holistic," which generally means that the healthcare practitioner considers the whole person, including physical, mental, emotional, and spiritual health. Some of these therapies are also known as "preventive," which means that the practitioner educates and

---

[43] Adapted from the NCCAM: **http://nccam.nih.gov/nccam/fcp/faq/index.html#what-is**.

treats the person to prevent health problems from arising, rather than treating symptoms after problems have occurred.

People use CAM treatments and therapies in a variety of ways. Therapies are used alone (often referred to as alternative), in combination with other alternative therapies, or in addition to conventional treatment (sometimes referred to as complementary). Complementary and alternative medicine, or "integrative medicine," includes a broad range of healing philosophies, approaches, and therapies. Some approaches are consistent with physiological principles of Western medicine, while others constitute healing systems with non-Western origins. While some therapies are far outside the realm of accepted Western medical theory and practice, others are becoming established in mainstream medicine.

Complementary and alternative therapies are used in an effort to prevent illness, reduce stress, prevent or reduce side effects and symptoms, or control or cure disease. Some commonly used methods of complementary or alternative therapy include mind/body control interventions such as visualization and relaxation, manual healing including acupressure and massage, homeopathy, vitamins or herbal products, and acupuncture.

What Are the Domains of Alternative Medicine?[44]

The list of CAM practices changes continually. The reason being is that these new practices and therapies are often proved to be safe and effective, and therefore become generally accepted as "mainstream" healthcare practices. Today, CAM practices may be grouped within five major domains: (1) alternative medical systems, (2) mind-body interventions, (3) biologically-based treatments, (4) manipulative and body-based methods, and (5) energy therapies. The individual systems and treatments comprising these categories are too numerous to list in this sourcebook. Thus, only limited examples are provided within each.

Alternative Medical Systems

Alternative medical systems involve complete systems of theory and practice that have evolved independent of, and often prior to, conventional biomedical approaches. Many are traditional systems of medicine that are

---

[44] Adapted from the NCCAM: **http://nccam.nih.gov/nccam/fcp/classify/index.html**

practiced by individual cultures throughout the world, including a number of venerable Asian approaches.

Traditional oriental medicine emphasizes the balance or disturbances of qi (pronounced chi) or vital energy in health and disease, respectively. Traditional oriental medicine consists of a group of techniques and methods including acupuncture, herbal medicine, oriental massage, and qi gong (a form of energy therapy). Acupuncture involves stimulating specific anatomic points in the body for therapeutic purposes, usually by puncturing the skin with a thin needle.

Ayurveda is India's traditional system of medicine. Ayurvedic medicine (meaning "science of life") is a comprehensive system of medicine that places equal emphasis on body, mind, and spirit. Ayurveda strives to restore the innate harmony of the individual. Some of the primary Ayurvedic treatments include diet, exercise, meditation, herbs, massage, exposure to sunlight, and controlled breathing.

Other traditional healing systems have been developed by the world's indigenous populations. These populations include Native American, Aboriginal, African, Middle Eastern, Tibetan, and Central and South American cultures. Homeopathy and naturopathy are also examples of complete alternative medicine systems.

Homeopathic medicine is an unconventional Western system that is based on the principle that "like cures like," i.e., that the same substance that in large doses produces the symptoms of an illness, in very minute doses cures it. Homeopathic health practitioners believe that the more dilute the remedy, the greater its potency. Therefore, they use small doses of specially prepared plant extracts and minerals to stimulate the body's defense mechanisms and healing processes in order to treat illness.

Naturopathic medicine is based on the theory that disease is a manifestation of alterations in the processes by which the body naturally heals itself and emphasizes health restoration rather than disease treatment. Naturopathic physicians employ an array of healing practices, including the following: diet and clinical nutrition, homeopathy, acupuncture, herbal medicine, hydrotherapy (the use of water in a range of temperatures and methods of applications), spinal and soft-tissue manipulation, physical therapies (such as those involving electrical currents, ultrasound, and light), therapeutic counseling, and pharmacology.

Mind-Body Interventions

Mind-body interventions employ a variety of techniques designed to facilitate the mind's capacity to affect bodily function and symptoms. Only a select group of mind-body interventions having well-documented theoretical foundations are considered CAM. For example, patient education and cognitive-behavioral approaches are now considered "mainstream." On the other hand, complementary and alternative medicine includes meditation, certain uses of hypnosis, dance, music, and art therapy, as well as prayer and mental healing.

Biological-Based Therapies

This category of CAM includes natural and biological-based practices, interventions, and products, many of which overlap with conventional medicine's use of dietary supplements. This category includes herbal, special dietary, orthomolecular, and individual biological therapies.

Herbal therapy employs an individual herb or a mixture of herbs for healing purposes. An herb is a plant or plant part that produces and contains chemical substances that act upon the body. Special diet therapies, such as those proposed by Drs. Atkins, Ornish, Pritikin, and Weil, are believed to prevent and/or control illness as well as promote health. Orthomolecular therapies aim to treat disease with varying concentrations of chemicals such as magnesium, melatonin, and mega-doses of vitamins. Biological therapies include, for example, the use of laetrile and shark cartilage to treat cancer and the use of bee pollen to treat autoimmune and inflammatory diseases.

Manipulative and Body-Based Methods

This category includes methods that are based on manipulation and/or movement of the body. For example, chiropractors focus on the relationship between structure and function, primarily pertaining to the spine, and how that relationship affects the preservation and restoration of health. Chiropractors use manipulative therapy as an integral treatment tool.

In contrast, osteopaths place particular emphasis on the musculoskeletal system and practice osteopathic manipulation. Osteopaths believe that all of the body's systems work together and that disturbances in one system may have an impact upon function elsewhere in the body. Massage therapists manipulate the soft tissues of the body to normalize those tissues.

Energy Therapies

Energy therapies focus on energy fields originating within the body (biofields) or those from other sources (electromagnetic fields). Biofield therapies are intended to affect energy fields (the existence of which is not yet experimentally proven) that surround and penetrate the human body. Some forms of energy therapy manipulate biofields by applying pressure and/or manipulating the body by placing the hands in or through these fields. Examples include Qi gong, Reiki and Therapeutic Touch.

Qi gong is a component of traditional oriental medicine that combines movement, meditation, and regulation of breathing to enhance the flow of vital energy (qi) in the body, improve blood circulation, and enhance immune function. Reiki, the Japanese word representing Universal Life Energy, is based on the belief that, by channeling spiritual energy through the practitioner, the spirit is healed and, in turn, heals the physical body. Therapeutic Touch is derived from the ancient technique of "laying-on of hands." It is based on the premises that the therapist's healing force affects the patient's recovery and that healing is promoted when the body's energies are in balance. By passing their hands over the patient, these healers identify energy imbalances.

Bioelectromagnetic-based therapies involve the unconventional use of electromagnetic fields to treat illnesses or manage pain. These therapies are often used to treat asthma, cancer, and migraine headaches. Types of electromagnetic fields which are manipulated in these therapies include pulsed fields, magnetic fields, and alternating current or direct current fields.

Can Alternatives Affect My Treatment?

A critical issue in pursuing complementary alternatives mentioned thus far is the risk that these might have undesirable interactions with your medical treatment. It becomes all the more important to speak with your doctor who can offer advice on the use of alternatives. Official sources confirm this view. Though written for women, we find that the National Women's Health Information Center's advice on pursuing alternative medicine is appropriate for patients of both genders and all ages.[45]

---

[45] Adapted from **http://www.4woman.gov/faq/alternative.htm** .

Is It Okay to Want Both Traditional and Alternative Medicine?

Should you wish to explore non-traditional types of treatment, be sure to discuss all issues concerning treatments and therapies with your healthcare provider, whether a physician or practitioner of complementary and alternative medicine. Competent healthcare management requires knowledge of both conventional and alternative therapies you are taking for the practitioner to have a complete picture of your treatment plan.

The decision to use complementary and alternative treatments is an important one. Consider before selecting an alternative therapy, the safety and effectiveness of the therapy or treatment, the expertise and qualifications of the healthcare practitioner, and the quality of delivery. These topics should be considered when selecting any practitioner or therapy.

Finding CAM References on Aphasia

Having read the previous discussion, you may be wondering which complementary or alternative treatments might be appropriate for aphasia. For the remainder of this chapter, we will direct you to a number of official sources which can assist you in researching studies and publications. Some of these articles are rather technical, so some patience may be required.

The Combined Health Information Database

For a targeted search, The Combined Health Information Database is a bibliographic database produced by health-related agencies of the Federal Government (mostly from the National Institutes of Health). This database is updated four times a year at the end of January, April, July, and October. Check the titles, summaries, and availability of CAM-related information by using the "Simple Search" option at the following Web site: **http://chid.nih.gov/simple/simple.html**. In the drop box at the top, select "Complementary and Alternative Medicine." Then type "aphasia" (or synonyms) in the second search box. We recommend that you select 100 "documents per page" and to check the "whole records" options. The following was extracted using this technique:

- **Homeopathy in Rehabilitation Medicine**

  Source: Physical Medicine and Rehabilitation Clinics of North America. 10(3): 705-727. August 1999.

Summary: This journal article discusses the role of homeopathy in rehabilitation medicine, emphasizing the individualized nature of homeopathic prescription. First, it presents background information about the homeopathic approach to care, the preparation of homeopathic medicines, the social and historical context for modern homeopathic practice, and the fundamental principles of homeopathic philosophy. Then, it provides a broad overview of epidemiological, laboratory, and clinical research in homeopathy, followed by a more focused review of homeopathic research in six areas of interest to physical medicine and rehabilitation: migraine headache, aphasia, fibromyalgia, head injury, vertigo, and sprains and soft tissue injury. It includes a case study illustrating the homeopathic treatment of mild traumatic brain injury. Finally, it discusses the prescription of combination homeopathic medicines and the single ingredients that make up these combination products. The article has 1 figure, 58 references, and a resource list.

- **Alternative Neurology (editorial)**

  Source: Archives of Neurology. 55(11): 1394-1395. November 1998.

  Summary: This editorial introduces the articles on alternative neurology included in this theme issue of the Archives. The issue presents seven articles and four editorials on such topics as the efficacy of the ketogenic diet for epilepsy (see AMJA01327), computer-assisted therapy for aphasia, ginkgo biloba for the treatment of Alzheimer's disease ([AD], see AMJA01326), vitamin therapy for patients with AD, and the most appropriate research designs for evaluating new alternative therapies for AD. This editorial has 12 references.

National Center for Complementary and Alternative Medicine

The National Center for Complementary and Alternative Medicine (NCCAM) of the National Institutes of Health (http://nccam.nih.gov) has created a link to the National Library of Medicine's databases to allow patients to search for articles that specifically relate to aphasia and complementary medicine. To search the database, go to the following Web site: **www.nlm.nih.gov/nccam/camonpubmed.html**. Select "CAM on PubMed." Enter "aphasia" (or synonyms) into the search box. Click "Go." The following references provide information on particular aspects of complementary and alternative medicine (CAM) that are related to aphasia:

- **A comparison of relaxation training and syntax stimulation for chronic nonfluent aphasia.**
  Author(s): Murray LL, Heather Ray A.

Source: Journal of Communication Disorders. 2001 January-April; 34(1-2): 87-113.

http://www.ncbi.nlm.nih.gov:80/entrez/query.fcgi?cmd=Retrieve&db=PubMed&list_uids=11322572&dopt=Abstract

- **An evaluation of short-term group therapy for people with aphasia.**
  Author(s): Brumfitt SM, Sheeran P.
  Source: Disability and Rehabilitation. 1997 June; 19(6): 221-30.
  http://www.ncbi.nlm.nih.gov:80/entrez/query.fcgi?cmd=Retrieve&db=PubMed&list_uids=9195139&dopt=Abstract

- **An on-line analysis of syntactic processing in Broca's and Wernicke's aphasia.**
  Author(s): Zurif E, Swinney D, Prather P, Solomon J, Bushell C.
  Source: Brain and Language. 1993 October; 45(3): 448-64.
  http://www.ncbi.nlm.nih.gov:80/entrez/query.fcgi?cmd=Retrieve&db=PubMed&list_uids=8269334&dopt=Abstract

- **Aphasia and dementia in childhood chronic lead encephalopathy: a curable form of acquired mental impairment.**
  Author(s): Romano C, Grossi-Bianchi ML.
  Source: Panminerva Medica. 1968 November; 10(11): 448-50. No Abstract Available.
  http://www.ncbi.nlm.nih.gov:80/entrez/query.fcgi?cmd=Retrieve&db=PubMed&list_uids=4974667&dopt=Abstract

- **Aphasia in bilinguals.**
  Author(s): Ramamurthi B, Chari P.
  Source: Acta Neurochir Suppl (Wien). 1993; 56: 59-66. Review.
  http://www.ncbi.nlm.nih.gov:80/entrez/query.fcgi?cmd=Retrieve&db=PubMed&list_uids=8498202&dopt=Abstract

- **Aphasia management considered in the context of the World Health Organization model of disablements.**
  Author(s): Rogers MA, Alarcon NB, Olswang LB.
  Source: Phys Med Rehabil Clin N Am. 1999 November; 10(4): 907-23, Ix. Review.
  http://www.ncbi.nlm.nih.gov:80/entrez/query.fcgi?cmd=Retrieve&db=PubMed&list_uids=10573715&dopt=Abstract

- **Aphasia rehabilitation resulting from melodic intonation therapy.**
  Author(s): Sparks R, Helm N, Albert M.

Source: Cortex. 1974 December; 10(4): 303-16. No Abstract Available.
http://www.ncbi.nlm.nih.gov:80/entrez/query.fcgi?cmd=Retrieve&db=PubMed&list_uids=4452250&dopt=Abstract

- **Aphasia: a care study.**
  Author(s): Stewart J, Creed J.
  Source: British Journal of Nursing (Mark Allen Publishing). 1994 March 10-23; 3(5): 226-9.
  http://www.ncbi.nlm.nih.gov:80/entrez/query.fcgi?cmd=Retrieve&db=PubMed&list_uids=8173267&dopt=Abstract

- **Comparative observations on the curative results of the treatment of central aphasia by puncturing the yumen point versus conventional acupuncture methods.**
  Author(s): Zhang Z, Zhao C.
  Source: J Tradit Chin Med. 1990 December; 10(4): 260-3. No Abstract Available.
  http://www.ncbi.nlm.nih.gov:80/entrez/query.fcgi?cmd=Retrieve&db=PubMed&list_uids=1703612&dopt=Abstract

- **CT scan lesion localization and response to melodic intonation therapy with nonfluent aphasia cases.**
  Author(s): Naeser MA, Helm-Estabrooks N.
  Source: Cortex. 1985 June; 21(2): 203-23.
  http://www.ncbi.nlm.nih.gov:80/entrez/query.fcgi?cmd=Retrieve&db=PubMed&list_uids=4028738&dopt=Abstract

- **Developmental aphasia: impaired rate of non-verbal processing as a function of sensory modality.**
  Author(s): Tallal P, Piercy M.
  Source: Neuropsychologia. 1973 October; 11(4): 389-98. No Abstract Available.
  http://www.ncbi.nlm.nih.gov:80/entrez/query.fcgi?cmd=Retrieve&db=PubMed&list_uids=4758181&dopt=Abstract

- **Drawing together: evaluation of a therapy programme for severe aphasia.**
  Author(s): Sacchett C, Byng S, Marshall J, Pound C.

Source: International Journal of Language & Communication Disorders / Royal College of Speech & Language Therapists. 1999 July-September; 34(3): 265-89.

http://www.ncbi.nlm.nih.gov:80/entrez/query.fcgi?cmd=Retrieve&db=PubMed&list_uids=10884902&dopt=Abstract

- **Effect of auditory prestimulation on naming in aphasia.**
  Author(s): Podraza BL, Darley FL.
  Source: Journal of Speech and Hearing Research. 1977 December; 20(4): 669-83.
  http://www.ncbi.nlm.nih.gov:80/entrez/query.fcgi?cmd=Retrieve&db=PubMed&list_uids=604681&dopt=Abstract

- **Effect of restricted cortical lesions on absolute thresholds and aphasia-like deficits in Japanese macaques.**
  Author(s): Heffner HE, Heffner RS.
  Source: Behav Neurosci. 1989 February; 103(1): 158-69.
  http://www.ncbi.nlm.nih.gov:80/entrez/query.fcgi?cmd=Retrieve&db=PubMed&list_uids=2923669&dopt=Abstract

- **Effects of hypnosis and imagery training on naming behavior in aphasia.**
  Author(s): Thompson CK, Hall HR, Sison CE.
  Source: Brain and Language. 1986 May; 28(1): 141-53.
  http://www.ncbi.nlm.nih.gov:80/entrez/query.fcgi?cmd=Retrieve&db=PubMed&list_uids=3719294&dopt=Abstract

- **Efficacy of acupuncture in the treatment of post-stroke aphasia.**
  Author(s): Zhang ZJ.
  Source: J Tradit Chin Med. 1989 June; 9(2): 87-9. No Abstract Available.
  http://www.ncbi.nlm.nih.gov:80/entrez/query.fcgi?cmd=Retrieve&db=PubMed&list_uids=2476636&dopt=Abstract

- **Electromagnetic articulography treatment for an adult with Broca's aphasia and apraxia of speech.**
  Author(s): Katz WF, Bharadwaj SV, Carstens B.
  Source: Journal of Speech, Language, and Hearing Research : Jslhr. 1999 December; 42(6): 1355-66.
  http://www.ncbi.nlm.nih.gov:80/entrez/query.fcgi?cmd=Retrieve&db=PubMed&list_uids=10599618&dopt=Abstract

- **Espousing melodic intonation therapy in aphasia rehabilitation: a case study.**
  Author(s): Goldfarb R, Bader E.
  Source: International Journal of Rehabilitation Research. Internationale Zeitschrift Fur Rehabilitationsforschung. Revue Internationale De Recherches De Readaptation. 1979; 2(3): 333-42.
  http://www.ncbi.nlm.nih.gov:80/entrez/query.fcgi?cmd=Retrieve&db=PubMed&list_uids=541150&dopt=Abstract

- **Family adjustment to aphasia.**
  Author(s): Davis GA.
  Source: Asha. 1990 November; 32(11): 63-4. No Abstract Available.
  http://www.ncbi.nlm.nih.gov:80/entrez/query.fcgi?cmd=Retrieve&db=PubMed&list_uids=2282087&dopt=Abstract

- **Memory disorders in aphasia--I. Auditory immediate recall.**
  Author(s): Gordon WP.
  Source: Neuropsychologia. 1983; 21(4): 325-39.
  http://www.ncbi.nlm.nih.gov:80/entrez/query.fcgi?cmd=Retrieve&db=PubMed&list_uids=6621861&dopt=Abstract

- **Optic aphasia, optic apraxia, and loss of dreaming.**
  Author(s): Pena-Casanova J, Roig-Rovira T, Bermudez A, Tolosa-Sarro E.
  Source: Brain and Language. 1985 September; 26(1): 63-71.
  http://www.ncbi.nlm.nih.gov:80/entrez/query.fcgi?cmd=Retrieve&db=PubMed&list_uids=2413956&dopt=Abstract

- **Recovery from nonfluent aphasia after melodic intonation therapy: a PET study.**
  Author(s): Belin P, Van Eeckhout P, Zilbovicius M, Remy P, Francois C, Guillaume S, Chain F, Rancurel G, Samson Y.
  Source: Neurology. 1996 December; 47(6): 1504-11.
  http://www.ncbi.nlm.nih.gov:80/entrez/query.fcgi?cmd=Retrieve&db=PubMed&list_uids=8960735&dopt=Abstract

- **Singing as therapy for apraxia of speech and aphasia: report of a case.**
  Author(s): Keith RL, Aronson AE.
  Source: Brain and Language. 1975 October; 2(4): 483-8. No Abstract Available.
  http://www.ncbi.nlm.nih.gov:80/entrez/query.fcgi?cmd=Retrieve&db=PubMed&list_uids=1218380&dopt=Abstract

- **Supporting Partners of People with Aphasia in Relationships and Cconversation (SPPARC).**
  Author(s): Lock S, Wilkinson R, Bryan K, Maxim J, Edmundson A, Bruce C, Moir D.
  Source: International Journal of Language & Communication Disorders / Royal College of Speech & Language Therapists. 2001; 36 Suppl: 25-30.
  http://www.ncbi.nlm.nih.gov:80/entrez/query.fcgi?cmd=Retrieve&db=PubMed&list_uids=11340791&dopt=Abstract

- **The case of the lawyer's lugubrious language: dysarthria plus primary progressive aphasia or dysarthria plus dementia?**
  Author(s): McNeil MR.
  Source: Seminars in Speech and Language. 1998; 19(1): 49-57; Quiz 57-8.
  http://www.ncbi.nlm.nih.gov:80/entrez/query.fcgi?cmd=Retrieve&db=PubMed&list_uids=9519392&dopt=Abstract

- **The effect of acupuncture on apoplectic aphasia.**
  Author(s): Zhang ZJ.
  Source: J Tradit Chin Med. 1989 September; 9(3): 169-70. No Abstract Available.
  http://www.ncbi.nlm.nih.gov:80/entrez/query.fcgi?cmd=Retrieve&db=PubMed&list_uids=2482395&dopt=Abstract

- **The effect of hyperbaric oxygen on communication function in adults with aphasia secondary to stroke.**
  Author(s): Sarno MT, Sarno JE, Diller L.
  Source: Journal of Speech and Hearing Research. 1972 March; 15(1): 42-8. No Abstract Available.
  http://www.ncbi.nlm.nih.gov:80/entrez/query.fcgi?cmd=Retrieve&db=PubMed&list_uids=5012810&dopt=Abstract

- **The interactive nature of auditory comprehension in aphasia.**
  Author(s): Pierce RS, DeStefano CC.
  Source: Journal of Communication Disorders. 1987 February; 20(1): 15-24.
  http://www.ncbi.nlm.nih.gov:80/entrez/query.fcgi?cmd=Retrieve&db=PubMed&list_uids=3819000&dopt=Abstract

- **The perception of stress as a semantic cue in aphasia.**
  Author(s): Blumstein S, Goodglass H.

Source: Journal of Speech and Hearing Research. 1972 December; 15(4): 800-6. No Abstract Available.
http://www.ncbi.nlm.nih.gov:80/entrez/query.fcgi?cmd=Retrieve&db=PubMed&list_uids=4672047&dopt=Abstract

- **The word. A neurologist's view on aphasia.**
  Author(s): Hurwitz LJ.
  Source: Gerontol Clin (Basel). 1971; 13(5): 307-19. No Abstract Available.
  http://www.ncbi.nlm.nih.gov:80/entrez/query.fcgi?cmd=Retrieve&db=PubMed&list_uids=5113982&dopt=Abstract

- **Treatment of acquired aphasia.**
  Author(s): Darley FL.
  Source: Adv Neurol. 1975; 7: 111-45. Review. No Abstract Available.
  http://www.ncbi.nlm.nih.gov:80/entrez/query.fcgi?cmd=Retrieve&db=PubMed&list_uids=1090128&dopt=Abstract

- **Upper extremity sensory feedback therapy in chronic cerebrovascular accident patients with impaired expressive aphasia and auditory comprehension.**
  Author(s): Balliet R, Levy B, Blood KM.
  Source: Archives of Physical Medicine and Rehabilitation. 1986 May; 67(5): 304-10.
  http://www.ncbi.nlm.nih.gov:80/entrez/query.fcgi?cmd=Retrieve&db=PubMed&list_uids=3518658&dopt=Abstract

- **Wh interrogative production in agrammatic aphasia: an experimental analysis of auditory-visual stimulation and direct-production treatment.**
  Author(s): Thompson CK, McReynolds LV.
  Source: Journal of Speech and Hearing Research. 1986 June; 29(2): 193-206.
  http://www.ncbi.nlm.nih.gov:80/entrez/query.fcgi?cmd=Retrieve&db=PubMed&list_uids=3724112&dopt=Abstract

Additional Web Resources

A number of additional Web sites offer encyclopedic information covering CAM and related topics. The following is a representative sample:

- Alternative Medicine Foundation, Inc.: **http://www.herbmed.org/**

- AOL: **http://search.aol.com/cat.adp?id=169&layer=&from=subcats**
- Chinese Medicine: **http://www.newcenturynutrition.com/**
- drkoop.com®:
  http://www.drkoop.com/InteractiveMedicine/IndexC.html
- Family Village: **http://www.familyvillage.wisc.edu/med_altn.htm**
- Google: **http://directory.google.com/Top/Health/Alternative/**
- Healthnotes: **http://www.thedacare.org/healthnotes/**
- Open Directory Project: **http://dmoz.org/Health/Alternative/**
- TPN.com: **http://www.tnp.com/**
- Yahoo.com: **http://dir.yahoo.com/Health/Alternative_Medicine/**
- WebMD®Health: **http://my.webmd.com/drugs_and_herbs**
- WellNet: **http://www.wellnet.ca/herbsa-c.htm**
- WholeHealthMD.com:
  http://www.wholehealthmd.com/reflib/0,1529,,00.html

The following is a specific Web list relating to aphasia; please note that any particular subject below may indicate either a therapeutic use, or a contraindication (potential danger), and does not reflect an official recommendation:

- **General Overview**

  Aphasia
  Source: Integrative Medicine Communications; www.onemedicine.com
  Hyperlink:
  http://www.drkoop.com/InteractiveMedicine/ConsLookups/Symptoms/aphasia.html

- **Chinese Medicine**

  Huatuo Zaizao Wan
  Alternative names: Huatuo Zaizao Pills
  Source: Pharmacopoeia Commission of the Ministry of Health, People's Republic of China

Hyperlink: http://www.newcenturynutrition.com/cgi-local/patent_herbs_db/db.cgi?db=default&Chinese=Huatuo%20Zaizao%20Wan&mh=10&sb=---&view_records=View+Records

Shixiang Fansheng Wan
Alternative names: Shixiang Fansheng Pills; Shixiang Fansheng Wan
(Shi Xiang Fan Sheng Wan)
Source: Pharmacopoeia Commission of the Ministry of Health, People's Republic of China
Hyperlink: http://www.newcenturynutrition.com/cgi-local/patent_herbs_db/db.cgi?db=default&Chinese=Shixiang%20Fansheng%20Wan&mh=10&sb=---&view_records=View+Records

- **Related Conditions**

Stroke
Source: Integrative Medicine Communications; www.onemedicine.com
Hyperlink:
http://www.drkoop.com/interactivemedicine/ConsConditions/Strokecc.html

General References

A good place to find general background information on CAM is the National Library of Medicine. It has prepared within the MEDLINEplus system an information topic page dedicated to complementary and alternative medicine. To access this page, go to the MEDLINEplus site at: **www.nlm.nih.gov/medlineplus/alternativemedicine.html.** This Web site provides a general overview of various topics and can lead to a number of general sources. The following additional references describe, in broad terms, alternative and complementary medicine (sorted alphabetically by title; hyperlinks provide rankings, information, and reviews at Amazon.com):

- **Alternative Medicine for Dummies** by James Dillard (Author); Audio Cassette, Abridged edition (1998), Harper Audio; ISBN: 0694520659; **http://www.amazon.com/exec/obidos/ASIN/0694520659/icongroupinterna**

- **Complementary and Alternative Medicine Secrets** by W. Kohatsu (Editor); Hardcover (2001), Hanley & Belfus; ISBN: 1560534400; **http://www.amazon.com/exec/obidos/ASIN/1560534400/icongroupinterna**

- **Dictionary of Alternative Medicine** by J. C. Segen; Paperback-2nd edition (2001), Appleton & Lange; ISBN: 0838516211; http://www.amazon.com/exec/obidos/ASIN/0838516211/icongroupinterna

- **Eat, Drink, and Be Healthy: The Harvard Medical School Guide to Healthy Eating** by Walter C. Willett, MD, et al; Hardcover - 352 pages (2001), Simon & Schuster; ISBN: 0684863375; http://www.amazon.com/exec/obidos/ASIN/0684863375/icongroupinterna

- **Encyclopedia of Natural Medicine, Revised 2nd Edition** by Michael T. Murray, Joseph E. Pizzorno; Paperback - 960 pages, 2nd Rev edition (1997), Prima Publishing; ISBN: 0761511571; http://www.amazon.com/exec/obidos/ASIN/0761511571/icongroupinterna

- **Integrative Medicine: An Introduction to the Art & Science of Healing** by Andrew Weil (Author); Audio Cassette, Unabridged edition (2001), Sounds True; ISBN: 1564558541; http://www.amazon.com/exec/obidos/ASIN/1564558541/icongroupinterna

- **New Encyclopedia of Herbs & Their Uses** by Deni Bown; Hardcover - 448 pages, Revised edition (2001), DK Publishing; ISBN: 078948031X; http://www.amazon.com/exec/obidos/ASIN/078948031X/icongroupinterna

- **Textbook of Complementary and Alternative Medicine** by Wayne B. Jonas; Hardcover (2003), Lippincott, Williams & Wilkins; ISBN: 0683044370; http://www.amazon.com/exec/obidos/ASIN/0683044370/icongroupinterna

For additional information on complementary and alternative medicine, ask your doctor or write to:

National Institutes of Health
National Center for Complementary and Alternative Medicine Clearinghouse
P. O. Box 8218
Silver Spring, MD 20907-8218

APPENDIX C. RESEARCHING NUTRITION

Overview

Since the time of Hippocrates, doctors have understood the importance of diet and nutrition to patients' health and well-being. Since then, they have accumulated an impressive archive of studies and knowledge dedicated to this subject. Based on their experience, doctors and healthcare providers may recommend particular dietary supplements to patients with aphasia. Any dietary recommendation is based on a patient's age, body mass, gender, lifestyle, eating habits, food preferences, and health condition. It is therefore likely that different patients with aphasia may be given different recommendations. Some recommendations may be directly related to aphasia, while others may be more related to the patient's general health. These recommendations, themselves, may differ from what official sources recommend for the average person.

In this chapter we will begin by briefly reviewing the essentials of diet and nutrition that will broadly frame more detailed discussions of aphasia. We will then show you how to find studies dedicated specifically to nutrition and aphasia.

Food and Nutrition: General Principles

What Are Essential Foods?

Food is generally viewed by official sources as consisting of six basic elements: (1) fluids, (2) carbohydrates, (3) protein, (4) fats, (5) vitamins, and (6) minerals. Consuming a combination of these elements is considered to be a healthy diet:

- **Fluids** are essential to human life as 80-percent of the body is composed of water. Water is lost via urination, sweating, diarrhea, vomiting, diuretics (drugs that increase urination), caffeine, and physical exertion.

- **Carbohydrates** are the main source for human energy (thermoregulation) and the bulk of typical diets. They are mostly classified as being either simple or complex. Simple carbohydrates include sugars which are often consumed in the form of cookies, candies, or cakes. Complex carbohydrates consist of starches and dietary fibers. Starches are consumed in the form of pastas, breads, potatoes, rice, and other foods. Soluble fibers can be eaten in the form of certain vegetables, fruits, oats, and legumes. Insoluble fibers include brown rice, whole grains, certain fruits, wheat bran and legumes.

- **Proteins** are eaten to build and repair human tissues. Some foods that are high in protein are also high in fat and calories. Food sources for protein include nuts, meat, fish, cheese, and other dairy products.

- **Fats** are consumed for both energy and the absorption of certain vitamins. There are many types of fats, with many general publications recommending the intake of unsaturated fats or those low in cholesterol.

Vitamins and minerals are fundamental to human health, growth, and, in some cases, disease prevention. Most are consumed in your diet (exceptions being vitamins K and D which are produced by intestinal bacteria and sunlight on the skin, respectively). Each vitamin and mineral plays a different role in health. The following outlines essential vitamins:

- **Vitamin A** is important to the health of your eyes, hair, bones, and skin; sources of vitamin A include foods such as eggs, carrots, and cantaloupe.

- **Vitamin B^1**, also known as thiamine, is important for your nervous system and energy production; food sources for thiamine include meat, peas, fortified cereals, bread, and whole grains.

- **Vitamin B^2**, also known as riboflavin, is important for your nervous system and muscles, but is also involved in the release of proteins from nutrients; food sources for riboflavin include dairy products, leafy vegetables, meat, and eggs.

- **Vitamin B^3**, also known as niacin, is important for healthy skin and helps the body use energy; food sources for niacin include peas, peanuts, fish, and whole grains

- **Vitamin B^6**, also known as pyridoxine, is important for the regulation of cells in the nervous system and is vital for blood formation; food sources for pyridoxine include bananas, whole grains, meat, and fish.

- **Vitamin B^{12}** is vital for a healthy nervous system and for the growth of red blood cells in bone marrow; food sources for vitamin B^{12} include yeast, milk, fish, eggs, and meat.

- **Vitamin C** allows the body's immune system to fight various diseases, strengthens body tissue, and improves the body's use of iron; food sources for vitamin C include a wide variety of fruits and vegetables.

- **Vitamin D** helps the body absorb calcium which strengthens bones and teeth; food sources for vitamin D include oily fish and dairy products.

- **Vitamin E** can help protect certain organs and tissues from various degenerative diseases; food sources for vitamin E include margarine, vegetables, eggs, and fish.

- **Vitamin K** is essential for bone formation and blood clotting; common food sources for vitamin K include leafy green vegetables.

- **Folic Acid** maintains healthy cells and blood and, when taken by a pregnant woman, can prevent her fetus from developing neural tube defects; food sources for folic acid include nuts, fortified breads, leafy green vegetables, and whole grains.

It should be noted that one can overdose on certain vitamins which become toxic if consumed in excess (e.g. vitamin A, D, E and K).

Like vitamins, minerals are chemicals that are required by the body to remain in good health. Because the human body does not manufacture these chemicals internally, we obtain them from food and other dietary sources. The more important minerals include:

- **Calcium** is needed for healthy bones, teeth, and muscles, but also helps the nervous system function; food sources for calcium include dry beans, peas, eggs, and dairy products.

- **Chromium** is helpful in regulating sugar levels in blood; food sources for chromium include egg yolks, raw sugar, cheese, nuts, beets, whole grains, and meat.

- **Fluoride** is used by the body to help prevent tooth decay and to reinforce bone strength; sources of fluoride include drinking water and certain brands of toothpaste.

- **Iodine** helps regulate the body's use of energy by synthesizing into the hormone thyroxine; food sources include leafy green vegetables, nuts, egg yolks, and red meat.

- **Iron** helps maintain muscles and the formation of red blood cells and certain proteins; food sources for iron include meat, dairy products, eggs, and leafy green vegetables.

- **Magnesium** is important for the production of DNA, as well as for healthy teeth, bones, muscles, and nerves; food sources for magnesium include dried fruit, dark green vegetables, nuts, and seafood.

- **Phosphorous** is used by the body to work with calcium to form bones and teeth; food sources for phosphorous include eggs, meat, cereals, and dairy products.

- **Selenium** primarily helps maintain normal heart and liver functions; food sources for selenium include wholegrain cereals, fish, meat, and dairy products.

- **Zinc** helps wounds heal, the formation of sperm, and encourage rapid growth and energy; food sources include dried beans, shellfish, eggs, and nuts.

The United States government periodically publishes recommended diets and consumption levels of the various elements of food. Again, your doctor may encourage deviations from the average official recommendation based on your specific condition. To learn more about basic dietary guidelines, visit the Web site: **http://www.health.gov/dietaryguidelines/**. Based on these guidelines, many foods are required to list the nutrition levels on the food's packaging. Labeling Requirements are listed at the following site maintained by the Food and Drug Administration: **http://www.cfsan.fda.gov/~dms/lab-cons.html**. When interpreting these requirements, the government recommends that consumers become familiar with the following abbreviations before reading FDA literature:[46]

- **DVs (Daily Values):** A new dietary reference term that will appear on the food label. It is made up of two sets of references, DRVs and RDIs.

- **DRVs (Daily Reference Values):** A set of dietary references that applies to fat, saturated fat, cholesterol, carbohydrate, protein, fiber, sodium, and potassium.

---

[46] Adapted from the FDA: **http://www.fda.gov/fdac/special/foodlabel/dvs.html**.

- **RDIs (Reference Daily Intakes):** A set of dietary references based on the Recommended Dietary Allowances for essential vitamins and minerals and, in selected groups, protein. The name "RDI" replaces the term "U.S. RDA."

- **RDAs (Recommended Dietary Allowances):** A set of estimated nutrient allowances established by the National Academy of Sciences. It is updated periodically to reflect current scientific knowledge.

What Are Dietary Supplements?[47]

Dietary supplements are widely available through many commercial sources, including health food stores, grocery stores, pharmacies, and by mail. Dietary supplements are provided in many forms including tablets, capsules, powders, gel-tabs, extracts, and liquids. Historically in the United States, the most prevalent type of dietary supplement was a multivitamin/mineral tablet or capsule that was available in pharmacies, either by prescription or "over the counter." Supplements containing strictly herbal preparations were less widely available. Currently in the United States, a wide array of supplement products are available, including vitamin, mineral, other nutrients, and botanical supplements as well as ingredients and extracts of animal and plant origin.

The Office of Dietary Supplements (ODS) of the National Institutes of Health is the official agency of the United States which has the expressed goal of acquiring "new knowledge to help prevent, detect, diagnose, and treat disease and disability, from the rarest genetic disorder to the common cold."[48] According to the ODS, dietary supplements can have an important impact on the prevention and management of disease and on the maintenance of health.[49] The ODS notes that considerable research on the effects of dietary supplements has been conducted in Asia and Europe where the use of plant products, in particular, has a long tradition. However, the

---

[47] This discussion has been adapted from the NIH:
http://ods.od.nih.gov/whatare/whatare.html.

[48] Contact: The Office of Dietary Supplements, National Institutes of Health, Building 31, Room 1B29, 31 Center Drive, MSC 2086, Bethesda, Maryland 20892-2086, Tel: (301) 435-2920, Fax: (301) 480-1845, E-mail: **ods@nih.gov**.

[49] Adapted from **http://ods.od.nih.gov/about/about.html**. The Dietary Supplement Health and Education Act defines dietary supplements as "a product (other than tobacco) intended to supplement the diet that bears or contains one or more of the following dietary ingredients: a vitamin, mineral, amino acid, herb or other botanical; or a dietary substance for use to supplement the diet by increasing the total dietary intake; or a concentrate, metabolite, constituent, extract, or combination of any ingredient described above; and intended for ingestion in the form of a capsule, powder, softgel, or gelcap, and not represented as a conventional food or as a sole item of a meal or the diet."

overwhelming majority of supplements have not been studied scientifically. To explore the role of dietary supplements in the improvement of health care, the ODS plans, organizes, and supports conferences, workshops, and symposia on scientific topics related to dietary supplements. The ODS often works in conjunction with other NIH Institutes and Centers, other government agencies, professional organizations, and public advocacy groups.

To learn more about official information on dietary supplements, visit the ODS site at **http://ods.od.nih.gov/whatare/whatare.html**. Or contact:

> The Office of Dietary Supplements
> National Institutes of Health
> Building 31, Room 1B29
> 31 Center Drive, MSC 2086
> Bethesda, Maryland 20892-2086
> Tel: (301) 435-2920
> Fax: (301) 480-1845
> E-mail: ods@nih.gov

Finding Studies on Aphasia

The NIH maintains an office dedicated to patient nutrition and diet. The National Institutes of Health's Office of Dietary Supplements (ODS) offers a searchable bibliographic database called the IBIDS (International Bibliographic Information on Dietary Supplements). The IBIDS contains over 460,000 scientific citations and summaries about dietary supplements and nutrition as well as references to published international, scientific literature on dietary supplements such as vitamins, minerals, and botanicals.[50] IBIDS is available to the public free of charge through the ODS Internet page: **http://ods.od.nih.gov/databases/ibids.html**.

After entering the search area, you have three choices: (1) IBIDS Consumer Database, (2) Full IBIDS Database, or (3) Peer Reviewed Citations Only. We recommend that you start with the Consumer Database. While you may not find references for the topics that are of most interest to you, check back periodically as this database is frequently updated. More studies can be

---

[50] Adapted from **http://ods.od.nih.gov**. IBIDS is produced by the Office of Dietary Supplements (ODS) at the National Institutes of Health to assist the public, healthcare providers, educators, and researchers in locating credible, scientific information on dietary supplements. IBIDS was developed and will be maintained through an interagency partnership with the Food and Nutrition Information Center of the National Agricultural Library, U.S. Department of Agriculture.

found by searching the Full IBIDS Database. Healthcare professionals and researchers generally use the third option, which lists peer-reviewed citations. In all cases, we suggest that you take advantage of the "Advanced Search" option that allows you to retrieve up to 100 fully explained references in a comprehensive format. Type "aphasia" (or synonyms) into the search box. To narrow the search, you can also select the "Title" field.

The following information is typical of that found when using the "Full IBIDS Database" when searching using "aphasia" (or a synonym):

- **A randomized, double-blind, placebo-controlled study of bromocriptine in nonfluent aphasia.**
  Author(s): Department of Behavioral Neurology, Raul Carrea Institute of Neurological Research, Buenos Aires, Argentina.
  Source: Sabe, L Salvarezza, F Garcia Cuerva, A Leiguarda, R Starkstein, S Neurology. 1995 December; 45(12): 2272-4 0028-3878

- **Acquired aphasia with convulsive disorder: a pervasive developmental disorder variant.**
  Author(s): Department of Pediatrics, New York Hospital--Cornell Medical Center, New York.
  Source: Nass, R Petrucha, D JChild-Neurol. 1990 October; 5(4): 327-8 0883-0738

- **An open-label trial of bromocriptine in nonfluent aphasia.**
  Author(s): Institute of Neurological Research Raul Carrea, Buenos Aires, Argentina.
  Source: Sabe, L Leiguarda, R Starkstein, S E Neurology. 1992 August; 42(8): 1637-8 0028-3878

- **An open-label trial of bromocriptine in nonfluent aphasia: a qualitative analysis of word storage and retrieval.**
  Author(s): Department of Neurology, University of South Florida College of Medicine, Tampa, 33612, USA. mgold@com1.med.usf.edu
  Source: Gold, M VanDam, D Silliman, E R Brain-Lang. 2000 September; 74(2): 141-56 0093-934X

- **Bromocriptine and speech therapy in non-fluent chronic aphasia after stroke.**
  Author(s): Department of Neurological Sciences, University of Roma La Sapienza, Italy.
  Source: Bragoni, M Altieri, M Di Piero, V Padovani, A Mostardini, C Lenzi, G L Neurol-Sci. 2000 February; 21(1): 19-22 1590-1874

- **Bromocriptine is ineffective in the treatment of chronic nonfluent aphasia.**
  Author(s): Department of Neurology, School of Medicine, Cukurova University, Balcali, Adana, Turkey.
  Source: Ozeren, A Sarica, Y Mavi, H Demirkiran, M Acta-Neurol-Belg. 1995 December; 95(4): 235-8 0300-9009

- **Bromocriptine treatment of nonfluent aphasia.**
  Author(s): Neurology Service, Edward Hines Jr. Veterans Affairs Hospital, Hines, IL 60141, USA.
  Source: Gupta, S R Mlcoch, A G Scolaro, C Moritz, T Neurology. 1995 December; 45(12): 2170-3 0028-3878

- **Bromocriptine-induced dystonia in patients with aphasia and hemiparesis.**
  Author(s): Raul Carrea Institute of Neurological Research, Fundacion para la Lucha contra las Enfermedades Neurologicas de la Infancia (FLENI), Buenos Aires, Argentina.
  Source: Leiguarda, R Merello, M Sabe, L Starkstein, S Neurology. 1993 November; 43(11): 2319-22 0028-3878

- **Comparative observations on the curative results of the treatment of central aphasia by puncturing the yumen point versus conventional acupuncture methods.**
  Author(s): 266th PLA Hospital.
  Source: Zhang, Z Zhao, C J-Tradit-Chin-Med. 1990 December; 10(4): 260-3 0254-6272

- **Corticosteroid-responsive postmalaria encephalopathy characterized by motor aphasia, myoclonus, and postural tremor.**
  Author(s): Department of Neurology, University Hospital of Geneva, Switzerland.
  Source: Schnorf, H Diserens, K Schnyder, H Chofflon, M Loutan, L Chaves, V Landis, T Arch-Neurol. 1998 March; 55(3): 417-20 0003-9942

- **Effects of bromocriptine in a patient with crossed nonfluent aphasia: a case report.**
  Author(s): Old Dominion University, Norfolk, VA, USA. sraymer@odu.edu
  Source: Raymer, A M Bandy, D Adair, J C Schwartz, R L Williamson, D J Gonzalez Rothi, L J Heilman, K M Arch-Phys-Med-Rehabil. 2001 January; 82(1): 139-44 0003-9993

- **Efficacy of acupuncture in the treatment of post-stroke aphasia.**
  Source: Zhang, Z J J-Tradit-Chin-Med. 1989 June; 9(2): 87-9 0254-6272

- **Low erythrocyte zinc content in acquired aphasia with convulsive disorder (Landau-Kleffner syndrome).**
  Source: Lerman Sagie, T Statter, M Lerman, P J-Child-Neurol. 1987 January; 2(1): 28-30 0883-0738

- **Motor aphasia due to prolonged hypoglycaemic coma in a patient with insulin-dependent diabetes mellitus.**
  Author(s): Department of Medicine, Kusatsu Branch Hospital, Gunma University Hospital, Japan.
  Source: Kurabayashi, H Kubota, K Tamura, K Akiba, T Shirakura, T J-Int-Med-Res. 1996 Nov-December; 24(6): 487-91 0300-0605

- **Pharmacotherapy for aphasia.**
  Author(s): Department of Neurology, Boston University Medical School, MA.
  Source: Albert, M L Bachman, D L Morgan, A Helm Estabrooks, N Neurology. 1988 June; 38(6): 877-9 0028-3878

- **The case of the lawyer's lugubrious language: dysarthria plus primary progressive aphasia or dysarthria plus dementia?**
  Author(s): Department of Communication Science and Disorders, University of Pittsburgh, PA 15260, USA.
  Source: McNeil, M R Semin-Speech-Lang. 1998; 19(1): 49-57; quiz 57-8 0734-0478

- **The effect of acupuncture on apoplectic aphasia.**
  Source: Zhang, Z J J-Tradit-Chin-Med. 1989 September; 9(3): 169-70 0254-6272

- **Transient motor aphasia and recurrent partial seizures in a child: language recovery upon seizure control.**
  Author(s): Neuropediatric Department, Hospital Saint Vincent de Paul, University Rene Descartes, Paris, France.
  Source: Jambaque, I Chiron, C Kaminska, A Plouin, P Dulac, O J-Child-Neurol. 1998 June; 13(6): 296-300 0883-0738

- **Treatment of acquired epileptic aphasia with the ketogenic diet.**
  Author(s): Pediatric Regional Epilepsy Program, Division of Neurology, The Children's Hospital of Philadelphia, PA 19104, USA. bergqvist@email.chop.edu
  Source: Bergqvist, A G Chee, C M Lutchka, L M Brooks Kayal, A R J-Child-Neurol. 1999 November; 14(11): 696-701 0883-0738

Federal Resources on Nutrition

In addition to the IBIDS, the United States Department of Health and Human Services (HHS) and the United States Department of Agriculture (USDA) provide many sources of information on general nutrition and health. Recommended resources include:

- healthfinder®, HHS's gateway to health information, including diet and nutrition:
  http://www.healthfinder.gov/scripts/SearchContext.asp?topic=238&page=0

- The United States Department of Agriculture's Web site dedicated to nutrition information: **www.nutrition.gov**

- The Food and Drug Administration's Web site for federal food safety information: **www.foodsafety.gov**

- The National Action Plan on Overweight and Obesity sponsored by the United States Surgeon General:
  http://www.surgeongeneral.gov/topics/obesity/

- The Center for Food Safety and Applied Nutrition has an Internet site sponsored by the Food and Drug Administration and the Department of Health and Human Services: **http://vm.cfsan.fda.gov/**

- Center for Nutrition Policy and Promotion sponsored by the United States Department of Agriculture: **http://www.usda.gov/cnpp/**

- Food and Nutrition Information Center, National Agricultural Library sponsored by the United States Department of Agriculture: **http://www.nal.usda.gov/fnic/**

- Food and Nutrition Service sponsored by the United States Department of Agriculture: **http://www.fns.usda.gov/fns/**

Additional Web Resources

A number of additional Web sites offer encyclopedic information covering food and nutrition. The following is a representative sample:

- AOL: **http://search.aol.com/cat.adp?id=174&layer=&from=subcats**

- Family Village: **http://www.familyvillage.wisc.edu/med_nutrition.html**

- Google: **http://directory.google.com/Top/Health/Nutrition/**

- Healthnotes: **http://www.thedacare.org/healthnotes/**

- Open Directory Project: **http://dmoz.org/Health/Nutrition/**

- Yahoo.com: **http://dir.yahoo.com/Health/Nutrition/**
- WebMD®Health: **http://my.webmd.com/nutrition**
- WholeHealthMD.com:
  http://www.wholehealthmd.com/reflib/0,1529,,00.html

Vocabulary Builder

The following vocabulary builder defines words used in the references in this chapter that have not been defined in previous chapters:

Bacteria: Unicellular prokaryotic microorganisms which generally possess rigid cell walls, multiply by cell division, and exhibit three principal forms: round or coccal, rodlike or bacillary, and spiral or spirochetal. [NIH]

Bromocriptine: A semisynthetic ergot alkaloid that is a dopamine D2 agonist. It suppresses prolactin secretion and is used to treat amenorrhea, galactorrhea, and female infertility, and has been proposed for Parkinson disease. [NIH]

Capsules: Hard or soft soluble containers used for the oral administration of medicine. [NIH]

Carbohydrate: An aldehyde or ketone derivative of a polyhydric alcohol, particularly of the pentahydric and hexahydric alcohols. They are so named because the hydrogen and oxygen are usually in the proportion to form water, $(CH_2O)n$. The most important carbohydrates are the starches, sugars, celluloses, and gums. They are classified into mono-, di-, tri-, poly- and heterosaccharides. [EU]

Cholesterol: The principal sterol of all higher animals, distributed in body tissues, especially the brain and spinal cord, and in animal fats and oils. [NIH]

Degenerative: Undergoing degeneration : tending to degenerate; having the character of or involving degeneration; causing or tending to cause degeneration. [EU]

Diarrhea: Passage of excessively liquid or excessively frequent stools. [NIH]

Insulin: A protein hormone secreted by beta cells of the pancreas. Insulin plays a major role in the regulation of glucose metabolism, generally promoting the cellular utilization of glucose. It is also an important regulator of protein and lipid metabolism. Insulin is used as a drug to control insulin-dependent diabetes mellitus. [NIH]

Iodine: A nonmetallic element of the halogen group that is represented by the atomic symbol I, atomic number 53, and atomic weight of 126.90. It is a nutritionally essential element, especially important in thyroid hormone synthesis. In solution, it has anti-infective properties and is used topically. [NIH]

Niacin: Water-soluble vitamin of the B complex occurring in various animal and plant tissues. Required by the body for the formation of coenzymes NAD and NADP. Has pellagra-curative, vasodilating, and antilipemic properties. [NIH]

Pediatrics: A medical specialty concerned with maintaining health and providing medical care to children from birth to adolescence. [NIH]

Potassium: An element that is in the alkali group of metals. It has an atomic symbol K, atomic number 19, and atomic weight 39.10. It is the chief cation in the intracellular fluid of muscle and other cells. Potassium ion is a strong electrolyte and it plays a significant role in the regulation of fluid volume and maintenance of the water-electrolyte balance. [NIH]

Riboflavin: Nutritional factor found in milk, eggs, malted barley, liver, kidney, heart, and leafy vegetables. The richest natural source is yeast. It occurs in the free form only in the retina of the eye, in whey, and in urine; its principal forms in tissues and cells are as FMN and FAD. [NIH]

Seizures: Clinical or subclinical disturbances of cortical function due to a sudden, abnormal, excessive, and disorganized discharge of brain cells. Clinical manifestations include abnormal motor, sensory and psychic phenomena. Recurrent seizures are usually referred to as EPILEPSY or "seizure disorder." [NIH]

Selenium: An element with the atomic symbol Se, atomic number 34, and atomic weight 78.96. It is an essential micronutrient for mammals and other animals but is toxic in large amounts. Selenium protects intracellular structures against oxidative damage. It is an essential component of glutathione peroxidase. [NIH]

Thyroxine: An amino acid of the thyroid gland which exerts a stimulating effect on thyroid metabolism. [NIH]

APPENDIX D. FINDING MEDICAL LIBRARIES

Overview

At a medical library you can find medical texts and reference books, consumer health publications, specialty newspapers and magazines, as well as medical journals. In this Appendix, we show you how to quickly find a medical library in your area.

Preparation

Before going to the library, highlight the references mentioned in this sourcebook that you find interesting. Focus on those items that are not available via the Internet, and ask the reference librarian for help with your search. He or she may know of additional resources that could be helpful to you. Most importantly, your local public library and medical libraries have Interlibrary Loan programs with the National Library of Medicine (NLM), one of the largest medical collections in the world. According to the NLM, most of the literature in the general and historical collections of the National Library of Medicine is available on interlibrary loan to any library. NLM's interlibrary loan services are only available to libraries. If you would like to access NLM medical literature, then visit a library in your area that can request the publications for you.[51]

---

[51] Adapted from the NLM: **http://www.nlm.nih.gov/psd/cas/interlibrary.html**

Finding a Local Medical Library

The quickest method to locate medical libraries is to use the Internet-based directory published by the National Network of Libraries of Medicine (NN/LM). This network includes 4626 members and affiliates that provide many services to librarians, health professionals, and the public. To find a library in your area, simply visit **http://nnlm.gov/members/adv.html** or call 1-800-338-7657.

Medical Libraries Open to the Public

In addition to the NN/LM, the National Library of Medicine (NLM) lists a number of libraries that are generally open to the public and have reference facilities. The following is the NLM's list plus hyperlinks to each library Web site. These Web pages can provide information on hours of operation and other restrictions. The list below is a small sample of libraries recommended by the National Library of Medicine (sorted alphabetically by name of the U.S. state or Canadian province where the library is located):[52]

- **Alabama:** Health InfoNet of Jefferson County (Jefferson County Library Cooperative, Lister Hill Library of the Health Sciences), **http://www.uab.edu/infonet/**

- **Alabama:** Richard M. Scrushy Library (American Sports Medicine Institute), **http://www.asmi.org/LIBRARY.HTM**

- **Arizona:** Samaritan Regional Medical Center: The Learning Center (Samaritan Health System, Phoenix, Arizona), **http://www.samaritan.edu/library/bannerlibs.htm**

- **California:** Kris Kelly Health Information Center (St. Joseph Health System), **http://www.humboldt1.com/~kkhic/index.html**

- **California:** Community Health Library of Los Gatos (Community Health Library of Los Gatos), **http://www.healthlib.org/orgresources.html**

- **California:** Consumer Health Program and Services (CHIPS) (County of Los Angeles Public Library, Los Angeles County Harbor-UCLA Medical Center Library) - Carson, CA, **http://www.colapublib.org/services/chips.html**

- **California:** Gateway Health Library (Sutter Gould Medical Foundation)

- **California:** Health Library (Stanford University Medical Center), **http://www-med.stanford.edu/healthlibrary/**

---

[52] Abstracted from **http://www.nlm.nih.gov/medlineplus/libraries.html**.

- **California:** Patient Education Resource Center - Health Information and Resources (University of California, San Francisco), **http://sfghdean.ucsf.edu/barnett/PERC/default.asp**

- **California:** Redwood Health Library (Petaluma Health Care District), **http://www.phcd.org/rdwdlib.html**

- **California:** San José PlaneTree Health Library, **http://planetreesanjose.org/**

- **California:** Sutter Resource Library (Sutter Hospitals Foundation), **http://go.sutterhealth.org/comm/resc-library/sac-resources.html**

- **California:** University of California, Davis. Health Sciences Libraries

- **California:** ValleyCare Health Library & Ryan Comer Cancer Resource Center (ValleyCare Health System), **http://www.valleycare.com/library.html**

- **California:** Washington Community Health Resource Library (Washington Community Health Resource Library), **http://www.healthlibrary.org/**

- **Colorado:** William V. Gervasini Memorial Library (Exempla Healthcare), **http://www.exempla.org/conslib.htm**

- **Connecticut:** Hartford Hospital Health Science Libraries (Hartford Hospital), **http://www.harthosp.org/library/**

- **Connecticut:** Healthnet: Connecticut Consumer Health Information Center (University of Connecticut Health Center, Lyman Maynard Stowe Library), **http://library.uchc.edu/departm/hnet/**

- **Connecticut:** Waterbury Hospital Health Center Library (Waterbury Hospital), **http://www.waterburyhospital.com/library/consumer.shtml**

- **Delaware:** Consumer Health Library (Christiana Care Health System, Eugene du Pont Preventive Medicine & Rehabilitation Institute), **http://www.christianacare.org/health_guide/health_guide_pmri_health _info.cfm**

- **Delaware:** Lewis B. Flinn Library (Delaware Academy of Medicine), **http://www.delamed.org/chls.html**

- **Georgia:** Family Resource Library (Medical College of Georgia), **http://cmc.mcg.edu/kids_families/fam_resources/fam_res_lib/frl.htm**

- **Georgia:** Health Resource Center (Medical Center of Central Georgia), **http://www.mccg.org/hrc/hrchome.asp**

- **Hawaii:** Hawaii Medical Library: Consumer Health Information Service (Hawaii Medical Library), **http://hml.org/CHIS/**

- **Idaho:** DeArmond Consumer Health Library (Kootenai Medical Center), **http://www.nicon.org/DeArmond/index.htm**

- **Illinois:** Health Learning Center of Northwestern Memorial Hospital (Northwestern Memorial Hospital, Health Learning Center), **http://www.nmh.org/health_info/hlc.html**

- **Illinois:** Medical Library (OSF Saint Francis Medical Center), **http://www.osfsaintfrancis.org/general/library/**

- **Kentucky:** Medical Library - Services for Patients, Families, Students & the Public (Central Baptist Hospital), **http://www.centralbap.com/education/community/library.htm**

- **Kentucky:** University of Kentucky - Health Information Library (University of Kentucky, Chandler Medical Center, Health Information Library), **http://www.mc.uky.edu/PatientEd/**

- **Louisiana:** Alton Ochsner Medical Foundation Library (Alton Ochsner Medical Foundation), **http://www.ochsner.org/library/**

- **Louisiana:** Louisiana State University Health Sciences Center Medical Library-Shreveport, **http://lib-sh.lsuhsc.edu/**

- **Maine:** Franklin Memorial Hospital Medical Library (Franklin Memorial Hospital), **http://www.fchn.org/fmh/lib.htm**

- **Maine:** Gerrish-True Health Sciences Library (Central Maine Medical Center), **http://www.cmmc.org/library/library.html**

- **Maine:** Hadley Parrot Health Science Library (Eastern Maine Healthcare), **http://www.emh.org/hll/hpl/guide.htm**

- **Maine:** Maine Medical Center Library (Maine Medical Center), **http://www.mmc.org/library/**

- **Maine:** Parkview Hospital, **http://www.parkviewhospital.org/communit.htm#Library**

- **Maine:** Southern Maine Medical Center Health Sciences Library (Southern Maine Medical Center), **http://www.smmc.org/services/service.php3?choice=10**

- **Maine:** Stephens Memorial Hospital Health Information Library (Western Maine Health), **http://www.wmhcc.com/hil_frame.html**

- **Manitoba, Canada:** Consumer & Patient Health Information Service (University of Manitoba Libraries), **http://www.umanitoba.ca/libraries/units/health/reference/chis.html**

- **Manitoba, Canada:** J.W. Crane Memorial Library (Deer Lodge Centre), **http://www.deerlodge.mb.ca/library/libraryservices.shtml**

- **Maryland:** Health Information Center at the Wheaton Regional Library (Montgomery County, Md., Dept. of Public Libraries, Wheaton Regional Library), **http://www.mont.lib.md.us/healthinfo/hic.asp**

- **Massachusetts:** Baystate Medical Center Library (Baystate Health System), **http://www.baystatehealth.com/1024/**

- **Massachusetts:** Boston University Medical Center Alumni Medical Library (Boston University Medical Center), **http://med-libwww.bu.edu/library/lib.html**

- **Massachusetts:** Lowell General Hospital Health Sciences Library (Lowell General Hospital), **http://www.lowellgeneral.org/library/HomePageLinks/WWW.htm**

- **Massachusetts:** Paul E. Woodard Health Sciences Library (New England Baptist Hospital), **http://www.nebh.org/health_lib.asp**

- **Massachusetts:** St. Luke's Hospital Health Sciences Library (St. Luke's Hospital), **http://www.southcoast.org/library/**

- **Massachusetts:** Treadwell Library Consumer Health Reference Center (Massachusetts General Hospital), **http://www.mgh.harvard.edu/library/chrcindex.html**

- **Massachusetts:** UMass HealthNet (University of Massachusetts Medical School), **http://healthnet.umassmed.edu/**

- **Michigan:** Botsford General Hospital Library - Consumer Health (Botsford General Hospital, Library & Internet Services), **http://www.botsfordlibrary.org/consumer.htm**

- **Michigan:** Helen DeRoy Medical Library (Providence Hospital and Medical Centers), **http://www.providence-hospital.org/library/**

- **Michigan:** Marquette General Hospital - Consumer Health Library (Marquette General Hospital, Health Information Center), **http://www.mgh.org/center.html**

- **Michigan:** Patient Education Resouce Center - University of Michigan Cancer Center (University of Michigan Comprehensive Cancer Center), **http://www.cancer.med.umich.edu/learn/leares.htm**

- **Michigan:** Sladen Library & Center for Health Information Resources - Consumer Health Information, **http://www.sladen.hfhs.org/library/consumer/index.html**

- **Montana:** Center for Health Information (St. Patrick Hospital and Health Sciences Center), **http://www.saintpatrick.org/chi/librarydetail.php3?ID=41**

- **National:** Consumer Health Library Directory (Medical Library Association, Consumer and Patient Health Information Section), **http://caphis.mlanet.org/directory/index.html**

- **National:** National Network of Libraries of Medicine (National Library of Medicine) - provides library services for health professionals in the United States who do not have access to a medical library, **http://nnlm.gov/**

- **National:** NN/LM List of Libraries Serving the Public (National Network of Libraries of Medicine), **http://nnlm.gov/members/**

- **Nevada:** Health Science Library, West Charleston Library (Las Vegas Clark County Library District), **http://www.lvccld.org/special_collections/medical/index.htm**

- **New Hampshire:** Dartmouth Biomedical Libraries (Dartmouth College Library), **http://www.dartmouth.edu/~biomed/resources.htmld/conshealth.htmld/**

- **New Jersey:** Consumer Health Library (Rahway Hospital), **http://www.rahwayhospital.com/library.htm**

- **New Jersey:** Dr. Walter Phillips Health Sciences Library (Englewood Hospital and Medical Center), **http://www.englewoodhospital.com/links/index.htm**

- **New Jersey:** Meland Foundation (Englewood Hospital and Medical Center), **http://www.geocities.com/ResearchTriangle/9360/**

- **New York:** Choices in Health Information (New York Public Library) - NLM Consumer Pilot Project participant, **http://www.nypl.org/branch/health/links.html**

- **New York:** Health Information Center (Upstate Medical University, State University of New York), **http://www.upstate.edu/library/hic/**

- **New York:** Health Sciences Library (Long Island Jewish Medical Center), **http://www.lij.edu/library/library.html**

- **New York:** ViaHealth Medical Library (Rochester General Hospital), **http://www.nyam.org/library/**

- **Ohio:** Consumer Health Library (Akron General Medical Center, Medical & Consumer Health Library), **http://www.akrongeneral.org/hwlibrary.htm**

- **Oklahoma:** Saint Francis Health System Patient/Family Resource Center (Saint Francis Health System), **http://www.sfh-tulsa.com/patientfamilycenter/default.asp**

- **Oregon:** Planetree Health Resource Center (Mid-Columbia Medical Center), **http://www.mcmc.net/phrc/**

- **Pennsylvania:** Community Health Information Library (Milton S. Hershey Medical Center), **http://www.hmc.psu.edu/commhealth/**

- **Pennsylvania:** Community Health Resource Library (Geisinger Medical Center), **http://www.geisinger.edu/education/commlib.shtml**

- **Pennsylvania:** HealthInfo Library (Moses Taylor Hospital), **http://www.mth.org/healthwellness.html**

- **Pennsylvania:** Hopwood Library (University of Pittsburgh, Health Sciences Library System), **http://www.hsls.pitt.edu/chi/hhrcinfo.html**

- **Pennsylvania:** Koop Community Health Information Center (College of Physicians of Philadelphia), **http://www.collphyphil.org/kooppg1.shtml**

- **Pennsylvania:** Learning Resources Center - Medical Library (Susquehanna Health System), **http://www.shscares.org/services/lrc/index.asp**

- **Pennsylvania:** Medical Library (UPMC Health System), **http://www.upmc.edu/passavant/library.htm**

- **Quebec, Canada:** Medical Library (Montreal General Hospital), **http://ww2.mcgill.ca/mghlib/**

- **South Dakota:** Rapid City Regional Hospital - Health Information Center (Rapid City Regional Hospital, Health Information Center), **http://www.rcrh.org/education/LibraryResourcesConsumers.htm**

- **Texas:** Houston HealthWays (Houston Academy of Medicine-Texas Medical Center Library), **http://hhw.library.tmc.edu/**

- **Texas:** Matustik Family Resource Center (Cook Children's Health Care System), **http://www.cookchildrens.com/Matustik_Library.html**

- **Washington:** Community Health Library (Kittitas Valley Community Hospital), **http://www.kvch.com/**

- **Washington:** Southwest Washington Medical Center Library (Southwest Washington Medical Center), **http://www.swmedctr.com/Home/**

APPENDIX E. YOUR RIGHTS AND INSURANCE

Overview

Any patient with aphasia faces a series of issues related more to the healthcare industry than to the medical condition itself. This appendix covers two important topics in this regard: your rights and responsibilities as a patient, and how to get the most out of your medical insurance plan.

Your Rights as a Patient

The President's Advisory Commission on Consumer Protection and Quality in the Healthcare Industry has created the following summary of your rights as a patient.[53]

Information Disclosure

Consumers have the right to receive accurate, easily understood information. Some consumers require assistance in making informed decisions about health plans, health professionals, and healthcare facilities. Such information includes:

- *Health plans.* Covered benefits, cost-sharing, and procedures for resolving complaints, licensure, certification, and accreditation status, comparable measures of quality and consumer satisfaction, provider network composition, the procedures that govern access to specialists and emergency services, and care management information.

---

[53]Adapted from Consumer Bill of Rights and Responsibilities:
http://www.hcqualitycommission.gov/press/cbor.html#head1.

- *Health professionals.* Education, board certification, and recertification, years of practice, experience performing certain procedures, and comparable measures of quality and consumer satisfaction.

- *Healthcare facilities.* Experience in performing certain procedures and services, accreditation status, comparable measures of quality, worker, and consumer satisfaction, and procedures for resolving complaints.

- *Consumer assistance programs.* Programs must be carefully structured to promote consumer confidence and to work cooperatively with health plans, providers, payers, and regulators. Desirable characteristics of such programs are sponsorship that ensures accountability to the interests of consumers and stable, adequate funding.

Choice of Providers and Plans

Consumers have the right to a choice of healthcare providers that is sufficient to ensure access to appropriate high-quality healthcare. To ensure such choice, the Commission recommends the following:

- *Provider network adequacy.* All health plan networks should provide access to sufficient numbers and types of providers to assure that all covered services will be accessible without unreasonable delay -- including access to emergency services 24 hours a day and 7 days a week. If a health plan has an insufficient number or type of providers to provide a covered benefit with the appropriate degree of specialization, the plan should ensure that the consumer obtains the benefit outside the network at no greater cost than if the benefit were obtained from participating providers.

- *Women's health services.* Women should be able to choose a qualified provider offered by a plan -- such as gynecologists, certified nurse midwives, and other qualified healthcare providers -- for the provision of covered care necessary to provide routine and preventative women's healthcare services.

- *Access to specialists.* Consumers with complex or serious medical conditions who require frequent specialty care should have direct access to a qualified specialist of their choice within a plan's network of providers. Authorizations, when required, should be for an adequate number of direct access visits under an approved treatment plan.

- *Transitional care.* Consumers who are undergoing a course of treatment for a chronic or disabling condition (or who are in the second or third trimester of a pregnancy) at the time they involuntarily change health plans or at a time when a provider is terminated by a plan for other than cause should be able to continue seeing their current specialty providers for up to 90 days (or through completion of postpartum care) to allow for transition of care.

- *Choice of health plans.* Public and private group purchasers should, wherever feasible, offer consumers a choice of high-quality health insurance plans.

Access to Emergency Services

Consumers have the right to access emergency healthcare services when and where the need arises. Health plans should provide payment when a consumer presents to an emergency department with acute symptoms of sufficient severity--including severe pain--such that a "prudent layperson" could reasonably expect the absence of medical attention to result in placing that consumer's health in serious jeopardy, serious impairment to bodily functions, or serious dysfunction of any bodily organ or part.

Participation in Treatment Decisions

Consumers have the right and responsibility to fully participate in all decisions related to their healthcare. Consumers who are unable to fully participate in treatment decisions have the right to be represented by parents, guardians, family members, or other conservators. Physicians and other health professionals should:

- Provide patients with sufficient information and opportunity to decide among treatment options consistent with the informed consent process.

- Discuss all treatment options with a patient in a culturally competent manner, including the option of no treatment at all.

- Ensure that persons with disabilities have effective communications with members of the health system in making such decisions.

- Discuss all current treatments a consumer may be undergoing.

- Discuss all risks, benefits, and consequences to treatment or nontreatment.

- Give patients the opportunity to refuse treatment and to express preferences about future treatment decisions.

- Discuss the use of advance directives -- both living wills and durable powers of attorney for healthcare -- with patients and their designated family members.

- Abide by the decisions made by their patients and/or their designated representatives consistent with the informed consent process.

Health plans, health providers, and healthcare facilities should:

- Disclose to consumers factors -- such as methods of compensation, ownership of or interest in healthcare facilities, or matters of conscience -- that could influence advice or treatment decisions.

- Assure that provider contracts do not contain any so-called "gag clauses" or other contractual mechanisms that restrict healthcare providers' ability to communicate with and advise patients about medically necessary treatment options.

- Be prohibited from penalizing or seeking retribution against healthcare professionals or other health workers for advocating on behalf of their patients.

Respect and Nondiscrimination

Consumers have the right to considerate, respectful care from all members of the healthcare industry at all times and under all circumstances. An environment of mutual respect is essential to maintain a quality healthcare system. To assure that right, the Commission recommends the following:

- Consumers must not be discriminated against in the delivery of healthcare services consistent with the benefits covered in their policy, or as required by law, based on race, ethnicity, national origin, religion, sex, age, mental or physical disability, sexual orientation, genetic information, or source of payment.

- Consumers eligible for coverage under the terms and conditions of a health plan or program, or as required by law, must not be discriminated against in marketing and enrollment practices based on race, ethnicity, national origin, religion, sex, age, mental or physical disability, sexual orientation, genetic information, or source of payment.

Confidentiality of Health Information

Consumers have the right to communicate with healthcare providers in confidence and to have the confidentiality of their individually identifiable healthcare information protected. Consumers also have the right to review and copy their own medical records and request amendments to their records.

Complaints and Appeals

Consumers have the right to a fair and efficient process for resolving differences with their health plans, healthcare providers, and the institutions that serve them, including a rigorous system of internal review and an independent system of external review. A free copy of the Patient's Bill of Rights is available from the American Hospital Association.[54]

Patient Responsibilities

Treatment is a two-way street between you and your healthcare providers. To underscore the importance of finance in modern healthcare as well as your responsibility for the financial aspects of your care, the President's Advisory Commission on Consumer Protection and Quality in the Healthcare Industry has proposed that patients understand the following "Consumer Responsibilities."[55] In a healthcare system that protects consumers' rights, it is reasonable to expect and encourage consumers to assume certain responsibilities. Greater individual involvement by the consumer in his or her care increases the likelihood of achieving the best outcome and helps support a quality-oriented, cost-conscious environment. Such responsibilities include:

- Take responsibility for maximizing healthy habits such as exercising, not smoking, and eating a healthy diet.

- Work collaboratively with healthcare providers in developing and carrying out agreed-upon treatment plans.

- Disclose relevant information and clearly communicate wants and needs.

- Use your health insurance plan's internal complaint and appeal processes to address your concerns.

- Avoid knowingly spreading disease.

---

[54] To order your free copy of the Patient's Bill of Rights, telephone 312-422-3000 or visit the American Hospital Association's Web site: **http://www.aha.org**. Click on "Resource Center," go to "Search" at bottom of page, and then type in "Patient's Bill of Rights." The Patient's Bill of Rights is also available from Fax on Demand, at 312-422-2020, document number 471124.

[55] Adapted from **http://www.hcqualitycommission.gov/press/cbor.html#head1**.

- Recognize the reality of risks, the limits of the medical science, and the human fallibility of the healthcare professional.

- Be aware of a healthcare provider's obligation to be reasonably efficient and equitable in providing care to other patients and the community.

- Become knowledgeable about your health plan's coverage and options (when available) including all covered benefits, limitations, and exclusions, rules regarding use of network providers, coverage and referral rules, appropriate processes to secure additional information, and the process to appeal coverage decisions.

- Show respect for other patients and health workers.

- Make a good-faith effort to meet financial obligations.

- Abide by administrative and operational procedures of health plans, healthcare providers, and Government health benefit programs.

Choosing an Insurance Plan

There are a number of official government agencies that help consumers understand their healthcare insurance choices.[56] The U.S. Department of Labor, in particular, recommends ten ways to make your health benefits choices work best for you.[57]

1. Your options are important. There are many different types of health benefit plans. Find out which one your employer offers, then check out the plan, or plans, offered. Your employer's human resource office, the health plan administrator, or your union can provide information to help you match your needs and preferences with the available plans. The more information you have, the better your healthcare decisions will be.

2. Reviewing the benefits available. Do the plans offered cover preventive care, well-baby care, vision or dental care? Are there deductibles? Answers to these questions can help determine the out-of-pocket expenses you may face. Matching your needs and those of your family members will result in the best possible benefits. Cheapest may not always be best. Your goal is high quality health benefits.

---

[56] More information about quality across programs is provided at the following AHRQ Web site:
http://www.ahrq.gov/consumer/qntascii/qnthplan.htm .
[57] Adapted from the Department of Labor:
http://www.dol.gov/dol/pwba/public/pubs/health/top10-text.html.

3. Look for quality. The quality of healthcare services varies, but quality can be measured. You should consider the quality of healthcare in deciding among the healthcare plans or options available to you. Not all health plans, doctors, hospitals and other providers give the highest quality care. Fortunately, there is quality information you can use right now to help you compare your healthcare choices. Find out how you can measure quality. Consult the U.S. Department of Health and Human Services publication "Your Guide to Choosing Quality Health Care" on the Internet at **www.ahcpr.gov/consumer**.

4. Your plan's summary plan description (SPD) provides a wealth of information. Your health plan administrator can provide you with a copy of your plan's SPD. It outlines your benefits and your legal rights under the Employee Retirement Income Security Act (ERISA), the federal law that protects your health benefits. It should contain information about the coverage of dependents, what services will require a co-pay, and the circumstances under which your employer can change or terminate a health benefits plan. Save the SPD and all other health plan brochures and documents, along with memos or correspondence from your employer relating to health benefits.

5. Assess your benefit coverage as your family status changes. Marriage, divorce, childbirth or adoption, and the death of a spouse are all life events that may signal a need to change your health benefits. You, your spouse and dependent children may be eligible for a special enrollment period under provisions of the Health Insurance Portability and Accountability Act (HIPAA). Even without life-changing events, the information provided by your employer should tell you how you can change benefits or switch plans, if more than one plan is offered. If your spouse's employer also offers a health benefits package, consider coordinating both plans for maximum coverage.

6. Changing jobs and other life events can affect your health benefits. Under the Consolidated Omnibus Budget Reconciliation Act (COBRA), you, your covered spouse, and your dependent children may be eligible to purchase extended health coverage under your employer's plan if you lose your job, change employers, get divorced, or upon occurrence of certain other events. Coverage can range from 18 to 36 months depending on your situation. COBRA applies to most employers with 20 or more workers and requires your plan to notify you of your rights. Most plans require eligible individuals to make their COBRA election within 60 days of the plan's notice. Be sure to follow up with your plan sponsor if you don't receive notice, and make sure you respond within the allotted time.

7. HIPAA can also help if you are changing jobs, particularly if you have a medical condition. HIPAA generally limits pre-existing condition exclusions to a maximum of 12 months (18 months for late enrollees). HIPAA also requires this maximum period to be reduced by the length of time you had prior "creditable coverage." You should receive a certificate documenting your prior creditable coverage from your old plan when coverage ends.

8. Plan for retirement. Before you retire, find out what health benefits, if any, extend to you and your spouse during your retirement years. Consult with your employer's human resources office, your union, the plan administrator, and check your SPD. Make sure there is no conflicting information among these sources about the benefits you will receive or the circumstances under which they can change or be eliminated. With this information in hand, you can make other important choices, like finding out if you are eligible for Medicare and Medigap insurance coverage.

9. Know how to file an appeal if your health benefits claim is denied. Understand how your plan handles grievances and where to make appeals of the plan's decisions. Keep records and copies of correspondence. Check your health benefits package and your SPD to determine who is responsible for handling problems with benefit claims. Contact PWBA for customer service assistance if you are unable to obtain a response to your complaint.

10. You can take steps to improve the quality of the healthcare and the health benefits you receive. Look for and use things like Quality Reports and Accreditation Reports whenever you can. Quality reports may contain consumer ratings -- how satisfied consumers are with the doctors in their plan, for instance-- and clinical performance measures -- how well a healthcare organization prevents and treats illness. Accreditation reports provide information on how accredited organizations meet national standards, and often include clinical performance measures. Look for these quality measures whenever possible. Consult "Your Guide to Choosing Quality Health Care" on the Internet at **www.ahcpr.gov/consumer**.

Medicare and Medicaid

Illness strikes both rich and poor families. For low-income families, Medicaid is available to defer the costs of treatment. The Health Care Financing Administration (HCFA) administers Medicare, the nation's largest health insurance program, which covers 39 million Americans. In the following pages, you will learn the basics about Medicare insurance as well as useful contact information on how to find more in-depth information about Medicaid.[58]

Who is Eligible for Medicare?

Generally, you are eligible for Medicare if you or your spouse worked for at least 10 years in Medicare-covered employment and you are 65 years old and a citizen or permanent resident of the United States. You might also qualify for coverage if you are under age 65 but have a disability or End-Stage Renal disease (permanent kidney failure requiring dialysis or transplant). Here are some simple guidelines:

You can get Part A at age 65 without having to pay premiums if:

- You are already receiving retirement benefits from Social Security or the Railroad Retirement Board.

- You are eligible to receive Social Security or Railroad benefits but have not yet filed for them.

- You or your spouse had Medicare-covered government employment.

If you are under 65, you can get Part A without having to pay premiums if:

- You have received Social Security or Railroad Retirement Board disability benefit for 24 months.

- You are a kidney dialysis or kidney transplant patient.

Medicare has two parts:

- Part A (Hospital Insurance). Most people do not have to pay for Part A.
- Part B (Medical Insurance). Most people pay monthly for Part B.

Part A (Hospital Insurance)

Helps Pay For: Inpatient hospital care, care in critical access hospitals (small facilities that give limited outpatient and inpatient services to people in rural areas) and skilled nursing facilities, hospice care, and some home healthcare.

---

[58] This section has been adapted from the Official U.S. Site for Medicare Information: **http://www.medicare.gov/Basics/Overview.asp**.

Cost: Most people get Part A automatically when they turn age 65. You do not have to pay a monthly payment called a premium for Part A because you or a spouse paid Medicare taxes while you were working.

If you (or your spouse) did not pay Medicare taxes while you were working and you are age 65 or older, you still may be able to buy Part A. If you are not sure you have Part A, look on your red, white, and blue Medicare card. It will show "Hospital Part A" on the lower left corner of the card. You can also call the Social Security Administration toll free at 1-800-772-1213 or call your local Social Security office for more information about buying Part A. If you get benefits from the Railroad Retirement Board, call your local RRB office or 1-800-808-0772. For more information, call your Fiscal Intermediary about Part A bills and services. The phone number for the Fiscal Intermediary office in your area can be obtained from the following Web site: **http://www.medicare.gov/Contacts/home.asp**.

Part B (Medical Insurance)

Helps Pay For: Doctors, services, outpatient hospital care, and some other medical services that Part A does not cover, such as the services of physical and occupational therapists, and some home healthcare. Part B helps pay for covered services and supplies when they are medically necessary.

Cost: As of 2001, you pay the Medicare Part B premium of $50.00 per month. In some cases this amount may be higher if you did not choose Part B when you first became eligible at age 65. The cost of Part B may go up 10% for each 12-month period that you were eligible for Part B but declined coverage, except in special cases. You will have to pay the extra 10% cost for the rest of your life.

Enrolling in Part B is your choice. You can sign up for Part B anytime during a 7-month period that begins 3 months before you turn 65. Visit your local Social Security office, or call the Social Security Administration at 1-800-772-1213 to sign up. If you choose to enroll in Part B, the premium is usually taken out of your monthly Social Security, Railroad Retirement, or Civil Service Retirement payment. If you do not receive any of the above payments, Medicare sends you a bill for your part B premium every 3 months. You should receive your Medicare premium bill in the mail by the 10th of the month. If you do not, call the Social Security Administration at 1-800-772-1213, or your local Social Security office. If you get benefits from the Railroad Retirement Board, call your local RRB office or 1-800-808-0772. For more information, call your Medicare carrier about bills and services. The phone number for the Medicare carrier in your area can be found at the following Web site: **http://www.medicare.gov/Contacts/home.asp**. You may have choices in how you get your healthcare including the Original Medicare Plan, Medicare Managed Care Plans (like HMOs), and Medicare Private Fee-for-Service Plans.

Medicaid

Medicaid is a joint federal and state program that helps pay medical costs for some people with low incomes and limited resources. Medicaid programs vary from state to state. People on Medicaid may also get coverage for nursing home care and outpatient prescription drugs which are not covered by Medicare. You can find more information about Medicaid on the HCFA.gov Web site at **http://www.hcfa.gov/medicaid/medicaid.htm**.

States also have programs that pay some or all of Medicare's premiums and may also pay Medicare deductibles and coinsurance for certain people who have Medicare and a low income. To qualify, you must have:

- Part A (Hospital Insurance),
- Assets, such as bank accounts, stocks, and bonds that are not more than $4,000 for a single person, or $6,000 for a couple, and
- A monthly income that is below certain limits.

For more information on these programs, look at the Medicare Savings Programs brochure, **http://www.medicare.gov/Library/PDFNavigation/PDFInterim.asp?Language=English&Type=Pub&PubID=10126**. There are also Prescription Drug Assistance Programs available. Find information on these programs which offer discounts or free medications to individuals in need at **http://www.medicare.gov/Prescription/Home.asp**.

NORD's Medication Assistance Programs

Finally, the National Organization for Rare Disorders, Inc. (NORD) administers medication programs sponsored by humanitarian-minded pharmaceutical and biotechnology companies to help uninsured or under-insured individuals secure life-saving or life-sustaining drugs.[59] NORD

---

[59] Adapted from NORD: **http://www.rarediseases.org/cgi-bin/nord/progserv#patient?id=rPIzL9oD&mv_pc=30**.

programs ensure that certain vital drugs are available "to those individuals whose income is too high to qualify for Medicaid but too low to pay for their prescribed medications." The program has standards for fairness, equity, and unbiased eligibility. It currently covers some 14 programs for nine pharmaceutical companies. NORD also offers early access programs for investigational new drugs (IND) under the approved "Treatment INDs" programs of the Food and Drug Administration (FDA). In these programs, a limited number of individuals can receive investigational drugs that have yet to be approved by the FDA. These programs are generally designed for rare diseases or disorders. For more information, visit **www.rarediseases.org**.

Additional Resources

In addition to the references already listed in this chapter, you may need more information on health insurance, hospitals, or the healthcare system in general. The NIH has set up an excellent guidance Web site that addresses these and other issues. Topics include:[60]

- Health Insurance:
  http://www.nlm.nih.gov/medlineplus/healthinsurance.html

- Health Statistics:
  http://www.nlm.nih.gov/medlineplus/healthstatistics.html

- HMO and Managed Care:
  http://www.nlm.nih.gov/medlineplus/managedcare.html

- Hospice Care: **http://www.nlm.nih.gov/medlineplus/hospicecare.html**

- Medicaid: **http://www.nlm.nih.gov/medlineplus/medicaid.html**

- Medicare: **http://www.nlm.nih.gov/medlineplus/medicare.html**

- Nursing Homes and Long-term Care:
  http://www.nlm.nih.gov/medlineplus/nursinghomes.html

- Patient's Rights, Confidentiality, Informed Consent, Ombudsman Programs, Privacy and Patient Issues:
  http://www.nlm.nih.gov/medlineplus/patientissues.html

---

[60] You can access this information at:
http://www.nlm.nih.gov/medlineplus/healthsystem.html.

APPENDIX F. MORE ON APHASIA RESEARCH

Overview[61]

Aphasia (uh-fay'-zhuh) is a communication disorder that can affect a person's ability to use and understand spoken or written words. It results from damage to the side of the brain dominant for language. For most people, this is the left side. Aphasia usually occurs suddenly and often results from a stroke or head injury, but it can also develop slowly because of a brain tumor, an infection, or dementia.

Types of Aphasia

There are many different classification systems for aphasia and many different types of aphasia within each system. Some systems are based primarily on the location of the lesion, while others are based solely on the person's behavior. One system adopted by the National Aphasia Association divides aphasia into two broad categories: fluent and non-fluent aphasia.

People with fluent aphasia have problems understanding spoken and written language. This type is also known as sensory, posterior, or Wernicke's aphasia.

People with non-fluent aphasia have difficulty communicating orally and in writing. This type of aphasia is also called motor, anterior, or Broca's aphasia. Within the non-fluent category is the most severe type, called global

---

[61] Adapted from The National Institute on Deafness and Other Communication Disorders (NIDCD): **http://www.nidcd.nih.gov/health/pubs_vsl/adultaphasia.htm** .

aphasia. People with this type have difficulty both expressing and understanding written and oral communication.

Aphasia Treatment

In general, treatment strives to improve a person's ability to communicate. The most effective treatment begins early in the recovery process and is maintained consistently over time. Major factors that influence the amount of improvement include the cause of the brain damage, the area of the brain that was damaged, the extent of the injury, and the person's general health.

Usually a speech-language pathologist works with other rehabilitation and medical professionals, such as physicians, nurses, neuropsychologists, occupational therapists, physical therapists, and social workers, as well as families, to provide a comprehensive evaluation and treatment plan for the person with aphasia.

Aphasia Research at NIDCD

The National Institute on Deafness and Other Communication Disorders (NIDCD) is one of the Institutes of the National Institutes of Health. The NIDCD supports and conducts biomedical and behavioral research and research training on normal and disordered processes of hearing, balance, smell, taste, voice, speech, and language. Currently supported aphasia research focuses on evaluating, characterizing, and treating the disorder, as well as on improving the understanding of the relationship between the language disorder and the brain.

New Approaches to Evaluation

Scientists are attempting to reveal the underlying problems that cause specific aphasia symptoms. The goal is to understand how injury to a particular brain structure impairs specific portions of a person's language process. The results could be useful in treating many types of aphasia, since the underlying cause can vary.

Other research is attempting to develop a model of sentence comprehension and production that can help provide a functional explanation for aphasia symptoms. These studies look at how difficulties in word representations and processes contribute to problems with sentence production and comprehension so that specific symptoms can be traced back to identifiable processing deficits. This would help focus treatment on the responsible word processes or representations.

New Approaches to Characterization

Since the same types of aphasia look different from one language to another, some scientists are attempting to distinguish between universal symptoms of the disorder and those that are language specific. Others are examining how people with aphasia maintain their knowledge of a language, but seem to have difficulty accessing that knowledge. Scientists are also comparing aspects of language that are at risk or are protected within and across language types and assessing the effect of stress on language expression in people without aphasia. These studies may help with the development of tests tailored to specific characteristics of individual languages and in clinical services to bilingual communities.

New Therapeutic Approaches

Pharmacotherapy is a new, experimental approach to treating aphasia. Some studies are testing how drugs can be used in combination with speech therapy to improve recovery of various language functions by increasing the task-related flow of activation in the left hemisphere of the brain. These studies indicate that drugs may help improve aphasia in acute stroke and as an adjuvant to language therapy in postacute and chronic aphasia.

Other treatment approaches use computers to improve the language abilities of people with aphasia. Studies have shown that computer-assisted therapy can help people with aphasia retrieve and produce verbs. People who have auditory problems perceiving the difference between phonemes can benefit from computers, which can be used for speech-therapeutic auditory discrimination exercises.

Researchers are also looking at how treatment of other cognitive deficits involving attention and memory can improve communication deficits.

A Closer Look at the Brain

To understand recovery processes in the brain, some researchers are attempting to use functional MRI (magnetic resonance imaging) to uncover the anatomical organization of the human brain regions involved in comprehending words and sentences. This type of research may improve understanding of how these areas reorganize after focal brain injury. The results could have implications for both the basic understanding of brain function and the diagnosis and treatment of neurological diseases.

About the Recent Research Series

This series is intended to inform health professionals, patients, and the public about progress in understanding the normal and disordered processes of human communication through recent advances made by NIDCD-supported scientists in each of the Institute's seven program areas: hearing, balance, smell, taste, voice, speech, and language.

If you have any other questions, contact:

NIDCD Information Clearinghouse
Toll-free: (800) 241-1044
Toll-free TTY: (800) 241-1055
Address: 1 Communication Avenue, Bethesda, MD 20892-3456
E-mail: nidcdinfo@nidcd.nih.gov
Internet: **www.nidcd.nih.gov**

For More Information

You can contact other groups as well for more information on aphasia:

Academy of Neurologic Communicative Disorders and Sciences
P.O. Box 26532
Minneapolis, MN 55426
E-mail: ancds@incnet.com
Internet: **www.duq.edu/ancds**

American Speech-Language-Hearing Association
10801 Rockville Pike
Rockville, MD 20852
Voice/TTY: (301) 897-5700
Toll-free: (800) 638-8255
Fax: (301) 897-7355
E-mail: actioncenter@asha.org
Internet: **www.asha.org**

Aphasia Hope Foundation
2436 West 137th Street
Leawood, KS 66224
Voice: (913) 402-8306
Toll-free: (866) 449-5804
Fax: (913) 402-8315
Internet: **www.aphasiahope.org**

National Aphasia Association
156 Fifth Avenue, Suite 707
New York, NY 10010
Voice: (212) 255-4329
Toll-free: (800) 922-4622
Fax: (212) 989-7777
E-mail: naa@aphasia.org
Internet: **www.aphasia.org**

ONLINE GLOSSARIES

The Internet provides access to a number of free-to-use medical dictionaries and glossaries. The National Library of Medicine has compiled the following list of online dictionaries:

- ADAM Medical Encyclopedia (A.D.A.M., Inc.), comprehensive medical reference: **http://www.nlm.nih.gov/medlineplus/encyclopedia.html**

- MedicineNet.com Medical Dictionary (MedicineNet, Inc.): **http://www.medterms.com/Script/Main/hp.asp**

- Merriam-Webster Medical Dictionary (Inteli-Health, Inc.): **http://www.intelihealth.com/IH/**

- Multilingual Glossary of Technical and Popular Medical Terms in Eight European Languages (European Commission) - Danish, Dutch, English, French, German, Italian, Portuguese, and Spanish: **http://allserv.rug.ac.be/~rvdstich/eugloss/welcome.html**

- On-line Medical Dictionary (CancerWEB): **http://www.graylab.ac.uk/omd/**

- Technology Glossary (National Library of Medicine) - Health Care Technology: **http://www.nlm.nih.gov/nichsr/ta101/ta10108.htm**

- Terms and Definitions (Office of Rare Diseases): **http://rarediseases.info.nih.gov/ord/glossary_a-e.html**

Beyond these, MEDLINEplus contains a very user-friendly encyclopedia covering every aspect of medicine (licensed from A.D.A.M., Inc.). The ADAM Medical Encyclopedia Web site address is **http://www.nlm.nih.gov/medlineplus/encyclopedia.html**. ADAM is also available on commercial Web sites such as Web MD (**http://my.webmd.com/adam/asset/adam_disease_articles/a_to_z/a**) and drkoop.com (**http://www.drkoop.com/**). Topics of interest can be researched by using keywords before continuing elsewhere, as these basic definitions and concepts will be useful in more advanced areas of research. You may choose to print various pages specifically relating to aphasia and keep them on file.

Online Dictionary Directories

The following are additional online directories compiled by the National Library of Medicine, including a number of specialized medical dictionaries and glossaries:

- Medical Dictionaries: Medical & Biological (World Health Organization): **http://www.who.int/hlt/virtuallibrary/English/diction.htm#Medical**

- MEL-Michigan Electronic Library List of Online Health and Medical Dictionaries (Michigan Electronic Library): **http://mel.lib.mi.us/health/health-dictionaries.html**

- Patient Education: Glossaries (DMOZ Open Directory Project): **http://dmoz.org/Health/Education/Patient_Education/Glossaries/**

- Web of Online Dictionaries (Bucknell University): **http://www.yourdictionary.com/diction5.html#medicine**

APHASIA GLOSSARY

The following is a complete glossary of terms used in this sourcebook. The definitions are derived from official public sources including the National Institutes of Health [NIH] and the European Union [EU]. After this glossary, we list a number of additional hardbound and electronic glossaries and dictionaries that you may wish to consult.

Accommodation: Adjustment, especially that of the eye for various distances. [EU]

Adjuvant: A substance which aids another, such as an auxiliary remedy; in immunology, nonspecific stimulator (e.g., BCG vaccine) of the immune response. [EU]

Agnosia: Loss of the ability to comprehend the meaning or recognize the importance of various forms of stimulation that cannot be attributed to impairment of a primary sensory modality. Tactile agnosia is characterized by an inability to perceive the shape and nature of an object by touch alone, despite unimpaired sensation to light touch, position, and other primary sensory modalities. [NIH]

Amphetamine: A powerful central nervous system stimulant and sympathomimetic. Amphetamine has multiple mechanisms of action including blocking uptake of adrenergics and dopamine, stimulation of release of monamines, and inhibiting monoamine oxidase. Amphetamine is also a drug of abuse and a psychotomimetic. The l- and the d,l-forms are included here. The l-form has less central nervous system activity but stronger cardiovascular effects. The d-form is dextroamphetamine. [NIH]

Aphasia: Defect or loss of the power of expression by speech, writing, or signs, or of comprehending spoken or written language, due to injury or disease of the brain centres. [EU]

Ataxia: Failure of muscular coordination; irregularity of muscular action. [EU]

Atypical: Irregular; not conformable to the type; in microbiology, applied specifically to strains of unusual type. [EU]

Audiology: The study of hearing and hearing impairment. [NIH]

Auditory: Pertaining to the sense of hearing. [EU]

Bacteria: Unicellular prokaryotic microorganisms which generally possess rigid cell walls, multiply by cell division, and exhibit three principal forms: round or coccal, rodlike or bacillary, and spiral or spirochetal. [NIH]

Bilateral: Having two sides, or pertaining to both sides. [EU]

Blindness: The inability to see or the loss or absence of perception of visual stimuli. This condition may be the result of eye diseases; optic nerve diseases; optic chiasm diseases; or brain diseases affecting the visual pathways or occipital lobe. [NIH]

Bromocriptine: A semisynthetic ergot alkaloid that is a dopamine D2 agonist. It suppresses prolactin secretion and is used to treat amenorrhea, galactorrhea, and female infertility, and has been proposed for Parkinson disease. [NIH]

Capsules: Hard or soft soluble containers used for the oral administration of medicine. [NIH]

Carbohydrate: An aldehyde or ketone derivative of a polyhydric alcohol, particularly of the pentahydric and hexahydric alcohols. They are so named because the hydrogen and oxygen are usually in the proportion to form water, $(CH2O)n$. The most important carbohydrates are the starches, sugars, celluloses, and gums. They are classified into mono-, di-, tri-, poly- and heterosaccharides. [EU]

Cardiogenic: Originating in the heart; caused by abnormal function of the heart. [EU]

Cerebral: Of or pertaining of the cerebrum or the brain. [EU]

Cerebrovascular: Pertaining to the blood vessels of the cerebrum, or brain. [EU]

Cholesterol: The principal sterol of all higher animals, distributed in body tissues, especially the brain and spinal cord, and in animal fats and oils. [NIH]

Chronic: Persisting over a long period of time. [EU]

Conduction: The transfer of sound waves, heat, nervous impulses, or electricity. [EU]

Confusion: Disturbed orientation in regard to time, place, or person, sometimes accompanied by disordered consciousness. [EU]

Cortex: The outer layer of an organ or other body structure, as distinguished from the internal substance. [EU]

Cues: Signals for an action; that specific portion of a perceptual field or pattern of stimuli to which a subject has learned to respond. [NIH]

Curative: Tending to overcome disease and promote recovery. [EU]

Degenerative: Undergoing degeneration : tending to degenerate; having the character of or involving degeneration; causing or tending to cause degeneration. [EU]

Dementia: An acquired organic mental disorder with loss of intellectual abilities of sufficient severity to interfere with social or occupational functioning. The dysfunction is multifaceted and involves memory, behavior, personality, judgment, attention, spatial relations, language, abstract thought, and other executive functions. The intellectual decline is usually progressive, and initially spares the level of consciousness. [NIH]

Diarrhea: Passage of excessively liquid or excessively frequent stools. [NIH]

Dizziness: An imprecise term which may refer to a sense of spatial disorientation, motion of the environment, or lightheadedness. [NIH]

Dominance: In genetics, the full phenotypic expression of a gene in both heterozygotes and homozygotes. [EU]

Dysarthria: Imperfect articulation of speech due to disturbances of muscular control which result from damage to the central or peripheral nervous system. [EU]

Dysphagia: Difficulty in swallowing. [EU]

Dystonia: Disordered tonicity of muscle. [EU]

Encephalopathy: Any degenerative disease of the brain. [EU]

Epidemiological: Relating to, or involving epidemiology. [EU]

Extremity: A limb; an arm or leg (membrum); sometimes applied specifically to a hand or foot. [EU]

Hemiplegia: Paralysis of one side of the body. [EU]

Hemorrhage: Bleeding or escape of blood from a vessel. [NIH]

Hyperbaric: Characterized by greater than normal pressure or weight; applied to gases under greater than atmospheric pressure, as hyperbaric oxygen, or to a solution of greater specific gravity than another taken as a standard of reference. [EU]

Individuality: Those psychological characteristics which differentiate individuals from one another. [NIH]

Infarction: 1. the formation of an infarct. 2. an infarct. [EU]

Insulin: A protein hormone secreted by beta cells of the pancreas. Insulin plays a major role in the regulation of glucose metabolism, generally promoting the cellular utilization of glucose. It is also an important regulator of protein and lipid metabolism. Insulin is used as a drug to control insulin-dependent diabetes mellitus. [NIH]

Intestinal: Pertaining to the intestine. [EU]

Iodine: A nonmetallic element of the halogen group that is represented by the atomic symbol I, atomic number 53, and atomic weight of 126.90. It is a nutritionally essential element, especially important in thyroid hormone synthesis. In solution, it has anti-infective properties and is used topically. [NIH]

Laryngectomy: Total or partial excision of the larynx. [NIH]

Larynx: An irregularly shaped, musculocartilaginous tubular structure, lined with mucous membrane, located at the top of the trachea and below the root of the tongue and the hyoid bone. It is the essential sphincter guarding the entrance into the trachea and functioning secondarily as the organ of voice. [NIH]

Lesion: Any pathological or traumatic discontinuity of tissue or loss of function of a part. [EU]

Lobe: A more or less well-defined portion of any organ, especially of the brain, lungs, and glands. Lobes are demarcated by fissures, sulci, connective tissue, and by their shape. [EU]

Localization: 1. the determination of the site or place of any process or lesion. 2. restriction to a circumscribed or limited area. 3. prelocalization. [EU]

Methotrexate: An antineoplastic antimetabolite with immunosuppressant properties. It is an inhibitor of dihydrofolate reductase and prevents the formation of tetrahydrofolate, necessary for synthesis of thymidylate, an essential component of DNA. [NIH]

Mobility: Capability of movement, of being moved, or of flowing freely. [EU]

Molecular: Of, pertaining to, or composed of molecules : a very small mass of matter. [EU]

Mutism: Inability or refusal to speak. [EU]

Neoplasms: New abnormal growth of tissue. Malignant neoplasms show a greater degree of anaplasia and have the properties of invasion and metastasis, compared to benign neoplasms. [NIH]

Neural: 1. pertaining to a nerve or to the nerves. 2. situated in the region of the spinal axis, as the neutral arch. [EU]

Neurology: A medical specialty concerned with the study of the structures, functions, and diseases of the nervous system. [NIH]

Neuropsychology: A branch of psychology which investigates the correlation between experience or behavior and the basic neurophysiological processes. The term neuropsychology stresses the dominant role of the nervous system. It is a more narrowly defined field than physiological psychology or psychophysiology. [NIH]

Neurosurgery: A surgical specialty concerned with the treatment of diseases and disorders of the brain, spinal cord, and peripheral and sympathetic nervous system. [NIH]

Niacin: Water-soluble vitamin of the B complex occurring in various animal and plant tissues. Required by the body for the formation of coenzymes NAD and NADP. Has pellagra-curative, vasodilating, and antilipemic properties. [NIH]

Norepinephrine: Precursor of epinephrine that is secreted by the adrenal medulla and is a widespread central and autonomic neurotransmitter. Norepinephrine is the principal transmitter of most postganglionic sympathetic fibers and of the diffuse projection system in the brain arising from the locus ceruleus. It is also found in plants and is used pharmacologically as a sympathomimetic. [NIH]

Otolaryngology: A surgical specialty concerned with the study and treatment of disorders of the ear, nose, and throat. [NIH]

Ototoxic: Having a deleterious effect upon the eighth nerve, or upon the organs of hearing and balance. [EU]

Overdose: 1. to administer an excessive dose. 2. an excessive dose. [EU]

Paralysis: Loss or impairment of motor function in a part due to lesion of the neural or muscular mechanism; also by analogy, impairment of sensory function (sensory paralysis). In addition to the types named below, paralysis is further distinguished as traumatic, syphilitic, toxic, etc., according to its cause; or as obturator, ulnar, etc., according to the nerve part, or muscle specially affected. [EU]

Parietal: 1. of or pertaining to the walls of a cavity. 2. pertaining to or located near the parietal bone, as the parietal lobe. [EU]

Pediatrics: A medical specialty concerned with maintaining health and providing medical care to children from birth to adolescence. [NIH]

Pharmacologic: Pertaining to pharmacology or to the properties and reactions of drugs. [EU]

Phobia: A persistent, irrational, intense fear of a specific object, activity, or situation (the phobic stimulus), fear that is recognized as being excessive or unreasonable by the individual himself. When a phobia is a significant source of distress or interferes with social functioning, it is considered a mental disorder; phobic disorder (or neurosis). In DSM III phobic disorders are subclassified as agoraphobia, social phobias, and simple phobias. Used as a word termination denoting irrational fear of or aversion to the subject indicated by the stem to which it is affixed. [EU]

Phonation: The process of producing vocal sounds by means of vocal cords vibrating in an expiratory blast of air. [NIH]

Posterior: Situated in back of, or in the back part of, or affecting the back or dorsal surface of the body. In lower animals, it refers to the caudal end of the body. [EU]

Postural: Pertaining to posture or position. [EU]

Potassium: An element that is in the alkali group of metals. It has an atomic symbol K, atomic number 19, and atomic weight 39.10. It is the chief cation in the intracellular fluid of muscle and other cells. Potassium ion is a strong electrolyte and it plays a significant role in the regulation of fluid volume and maintenance of the water-electrolyte balance. [NIH]

Prejudice: A preconceived judgment made without adequate evidence and not easily alterable by presentation of contrary evidence. [NIH]

Progressive: Advancing; going forward; going from bad to worse; increasing in scope or severity. [EU]

Prosthesis: An artificial substitute for a missing body part, such as an arm or leg, eye or tooth, used for functional or cosmetic reasons, or both. [EU]

Psychogenic: Produced or caused by psychic or mental factors rather than organic factors. [EU]

Psychology: The science dealing with the study of mental processes and behavior in man and animals. [NIH]

Remission: A diminution or abatement of the symptoms of a disease; also the period during which such diminution occurs. [EU]

Riboflavin: Nutritional factor found in milk, eggs, malted barley, liver, kidney, heart, and leafy vegetables. The richest natural source is yeast. It occurs in the free form only in the retina of the eye, in whey, and in urine; its principal forms in tissues and cells are as FMN and FAD. [NIH]

Rifabutin: A broad-spectrum antibiotic that is being used as prophylaxis against disseminated Mycobacterium avium complex infection in HIV-positive patients. [NIH]

Seizures: Clinical or subclinical disturbances of cortical function due to a sudden, abnormal, excessive, and disorganized discharge of brain cells. Clinical manifestations include abnormal motor, sensory and psychic phenomena. Recurrent seizures are usually referred to as epilepsy or "seizure disorder." [NIH]

Selenium: An element with the atomic symbol Se, atomic number 34, and atomic weight 78.96. It is an essential micronutrient for mammals and other animals but is toxic in large amounts. Selenium protects intracellular structures against oxidative damage. It is an essential component of glutathione peroxidase. [NIH]

Semantics: The relationships between symbols and their meanings. [NIH]

Shame: An emotional attitude excited by realization of a shortcoming or impropriety. [NIH]

Skull: The skeleton of the head including the bones of the face and the bones enclosing the brain. [NIH]

Socialization: The training or molding of an individual through various relationships, educational agencies, and social controls, which enables him to become a member of a particular society. [NIH]

Spasmodic: Of the nature of a spasm. [EU]

Symptomatology: 1. that branch of medicine with treats of symptoms; the systematic discussion of symptoms. 2. the combined symptoms of a disease. [EU]

Thermoregulation: Heat regulation. [EU]

Thrombosis: The formation, development, or presence of a thrombus. [EU]

Thyroxine: An amino acid of the thyroid gland which exerts a stimulating effect on thyroid metabolism. [NIH]

Tinnitus: A noise in the ears, as ringing, buzzing, roaring, clicking, etc. Such sounds may at times be heard by others than the patient. [EU]

Tomography: The recording of internal body images at a predetermined plane by means of the tomograph; called also body section roentgenography. [EU]

Tone: 1. the normal degree of vigour and tension; in muscle, the resistance to passive elongation or stretch; tonus. 2. a particular quality of sound or of voice. 3. to make permanent, or to change, the colour of silver stain by chemical treatment, usually with a heavy metal. [EU]

Toxicity: The quality of being poisonous, especially the degree of virulence of a toxic microbe or of a poison. [EU]

Vertigo: An illusion of movement; a sensation as if the external world were revolving around the patient (objective vertigo) or as if he himself were revolving in space (subjective vertigo). The term is sometimes erroneously used to mean any form of dizziness. [EU]

Vestibular: Pertaining to or toward a vestibule. In dental anatomy, used to refer to the tooth surface directed toward the vestibule of the mouth. [EU]

General Dictionaries and Glossaries

While the above glossary is essentially complete, the dictionaries listed here cover virtually all aspects of medicine, from basic words and phrases to more advanced terms (sorted alphabetically by title; hyperlinks provide rankings, information and reviews at Amazon.com):

- **Dictionary of Medical Acronymns & Abbreviations** by Stanley Jablonski (Editor), Paperback, 4th edition (2001), Lippincott Williams & Wilkins Publishers, ISBN: 1560534605, **http://www.amazon.com/exec/obidos/ASIN/1560534605/icongroupinterna**

- **Dictionary of Medical Terms : For the Nonmedical Person (Dictionary of Medical Terms for the Nonmedical Person, Ed 4)** by Mikel A. Rothenberg, M.D, et al, Paperback - 544 pages, 4th edition (2000), Barrons Educational

Series, ISBN: 0764112015,
http://www.amazon.com/exec/obidos/ASIN/0764112015/icongroupinterna

- **A Dictionary of the History of Medicine** by A. Sebastian, CD-Rom edition (2001), CRC Press-Parthenon Publishers, ISBN: 185070368X, http://www.amazon.com/exec/obidos/ASIN/185070368X/icongroupinterna

- **Dorland's Illustrated Medical Dictionary (Standard Version)** by Dorland, et al, Hardcover - 2088 pages, 29th edition (2000), W B Saunders Co, ISBN: 0721662544, http://www.amazon.com/exec/obidos/ASIN/0721662544/icongroupinterna

- **Dorland's Electronic Medical Dictionary** by Dorland, et al, Software, 29th Book & CD-Rom edition (2000), Harcourt Health Sciences, ISBN: 0721694934, http://www.amazon.com/exec/obidos/ASIN/0721694934/icongroupinterna

- **Dorland's Pocket Medical Dictionary (Dorland's Pocket Medical Dictionary, 26th Ed)** Hardcover - 912 pages, 26th edition (2001), W B Saunders Co, ISBN: 0721682812, http://www.amazon.com/exec/obidos/ASIN/0721682812/icongroupinterna /103-4193558-7304618

- **Melloni's Illustrated Medical Dictionary (Melloni's Illustrated Medical Dictionary, 4th Ed)** by Melloni, Hardcover, 4th edition (2001), CRC Press-Parthenon Publishers, ISBN: 85070094X, http://www.amazon.com/exec/obidos/ASIN/85070094X/icongroupinterna

- **Stedman's Electronic Medical Dictionary Version 5.0 (CD-ROM for Windows and Macintosh, Individual)** by Stedmans, CD-ROM edition (2000), Lippincott Williams & Wilkins Publishers, ISBN: 0781726328, http://www.amazon.com/exec/obidos/ASIN/0781726328/icongroupinterna

- **Stedman's Medical Dictionary** by Thomas Lathrop Stedman, Hardcover - 2098 pages, 27th edition (2000), Lippincott, Williams & Wilkins, ISBN: 068340007X, http://www.amazon.com/exec/obidos/ASIN/068340007X/icongroupinterna

- **Tabers Cyclopedic Medical Dictionary (Thumb Index)** by Donald Venes (Editor), et al, Hardcover - 2439 pages, 19th edition (2001), F A Davis Co, ISBN: 0803606540, http://www.amazon.com/exec/obidos/ASIN/0803606540/icongroupinterna

INDEX

Printed in the United States
20407LVS00001B/127

9 780597 831775